THE COMPLETE

KETO

BOOK FOR BEGINNERS

2021-2022

The Ultimate Beginners Keto Diet Cookbook
with Quick and Healthy 300 Low-Carb Recipes
Incl. 5 Week Weight Loss Plan

ISBN: 9798588010382

Table of Contents

INTRODUCTION 7

What is Keto Diet? 7
How does the keto diet work? 7
Benefits of keto diet? 8
What to Eat on a Keto Diet? 8
Healthy Fats 9
What can I eat? 9
What food can you eat on the Keto Diet? 10
What food can't you eat on Keto Diet? 10
What foods should you limit on Keto Diet? 10
How much does Keto Diet cost? 10
Does Keto Diet have any health risks? 10
Recipe Notes 10

28-DAYS KETO DIET MEALPLAN 11

First Week Meal Plan 12
Second Week Meal Plan 13
Third Week Meal Plan 14
Fourth Week Meal Plan 15

KETO BREAKFAST RECIPES 16

1.   Bulletproof Coffee 16
2.   Keto Butter Coffee 16
3.   Keto Boosted Coffee 16
4.   Keto Coffee Recipe 16
5.   Coconut oil Coffee 16
6.   Cabbage Hash Browns 17
7.   Omelet-Stuffed Peppers 17
8.   Scrambled eggs with basil 17
9.   Baked Eggs 18
10. Classic Bacon and eggs 18
11. Mexican scrambled eggs 18
12. Keto English Muffins 18
13. Seed & Nut Granola 19
14. Keto Oatmeal 19
15. Low-Carb Baked Eggs 19
16. Mexican egg roll 19
17. Keto Chia Pudding 20
18. Keto egg muffins 20
19. Fried Tomatoes 20
20. Beef and Green Beans 20
21. Egg and Ham Rolls 21
22. Blueberry Smoothie 21
23. Cheese Omelette 21
24. Spinach & Eggs 21
25. Bacon & Egg 22
26. Egg Medley Muffins 22
27. Cream Cheese Pancakes 22
28. Cheese Egg Wrap 22
29. Soldiers & Egg 23
30. Green Smoothie 23
31. Bacon Muffins 23
32. Avocado Sandwich 23

33. Breakfast Porridge 24
34. Scrambled Eggs 24
35. Avocado Coconut Milk 24
36. Fried Avocados 24
37. Veggie breakfast bakes 24
38. Cauliflower Hash 25
39. Butter Breakfast Balls 25
40. Keto deviled eggs 25
41. Tuna & Spinach Mix 26
42. Keto mushroom omelet 26
43. Almond Butter Choco 26
44. Fried Halloumi Cheese 26
45. Tomato baked eggs 27
46. Chives Egg Muffins 27
47. Filling Veg Soup 27
48. Turkey Wrap 28
49. Oven-Baked Brie Cheese 28
50. Keto cheese omelet 28
51. Keto smoked salmon 28
52. Keto Breakfast Burrito 29
53. Baked Broccoli Bites 29
54. Keto breakfast sandwich 29
55. Pancake Recipe 29
56. Keto Breakfast 30
57. Cheese & Bacon 30
58. Buttered Cabbage 30
59. Bacon & Spinach Bake 31
60. Cauliflower Medley 31
61. Olive Feast 31
62. Lime Pancakes 31
63. Keto Crepes Recipe 32
64. Wraps with Avocado 32
65. Peanut Butter Cookies 32
66. Bacon Cheddar Egg Cups 33
67. Broccoli and Cheddar 33
68. Strawberry Fat Bombs 33
69. Buffalo Chicken 33
70. Simple keto breakfast 34
71. Keto Breakfast Cake 34
72. Ham and Cheddar 34
73. Keto Breakfast Bake 35
74. Bacon Egg and Cheese 35
75. Keto Kimchi 35
76. Breakfast Fat Bombs 36
77. Breakfast Cookies 36
78. Breakfast Casserole 36
79. Egg Breakfast Wraps 37
80. Breakfast Sandwich 37
81. Breakfast Scramble 38
82. Low-Carb Keto 38
83. Keto Breakfast Pockets 38
84. Breakfast Bowl 39
85. Keto Tasty Casserole 39
86. Bacon Cheddar Keto 39
87. Chia Seeds Bread 40
88. Coconut Bread 40

89.	Carb-Free Bread	40
90.	Bacon and Avocado	41
91.	Keto Scrambled Eggs	41
92.	Keto Egg Wraps	41
93.	Keto Breakfast Muffins	42
94.	Sheet Pan Breakfast	42
95.	Bacon Egg and Cheese	42
96.	Egg & Sausage Breakfast	42
97.	Bacon & Broccoli Wrap	43
98.	Coconut Milk Shake	43
99.	Strawberry Pancakes	43
100.	Coconut Porridge	44

KETO LUNCH RECIPES 44

101.	Creamy Garlic Chicken	44
102.	Garlic Butter Steak	44
103.	Keto Guacamole	45
104.	Spicy Shrimp	45
105.	Tomatoes and Cheese	45
106.	Keto Egg Loaf	45
107.	Chewy Coconut Chunks	46
108.	Keto Carrot Cake	46
109.	Mozzarella Chicken	46
110.	Almond & Vanilla Keto	47
111.	Garlic Shrimp Zoodles	47
112.	Garlic Gnocchi	47
113.	Tangy & Tasty BBQ Pork	48
114.	Zucchini Pizza Boats	48
115.	Keto chicken enchilada	49
116.	Sassy Pork Stir-fry	49
117.	Shrimp & Sausage	49
118.	Keto Chili Kicker	50
119.	Salmon Lemon Sauce	50
120.	Coconut Chicken Curry	51
121.	Luscious Cheesy Choice	51
122.	Chicken Lettuce Wraps	52
123.	Healthy Lunchtime Ham	52
124.	Pancetta & Onion	52
125.	Hot & Spicy Chicken	53
126.	Cheesy Chicken Chunks	53
127.	Chunky Salsa Tacos	53
128.	Creamy Avocado	54
129.	Meatballs & Squash	54
130.	Spain Cheesy-Meat	54
131.	Cloud Nine BLT	55
132.	Pepperoni Pizza	55
133.	Cauliflower Cheese Bake	55
134.	Greek Salad	56
135.	Avocado Egg Salad	56
136.	Breakfast Mushroom	56
137.	Cauliflower Hash	57
138.	Baked Egg Banquet	57
139.	Cheese & Onion	57
140.	Shredded with Chicken	57
141.	Paleo Lamb Meatballs	58
142.	Carob Avocado Mousse	58
143.	Egg & Bacon Sandwich	58
144.	Baked Jalapeno Poppers	59
145.	Cheeseburger Frittata	59
146.	Keto Bread in a Mug	59
147.	Charming Cream Cheese	60
148.	Breakfast Casserole	60
149.	Bacon & Avocado	60
150.	Cheesy Chicken Fritters	61
151.	Garlic Butter Chicken	61
152.	Antipasto Salad Recipe	61
153.	Turkey Basil-Mayo	61
154.	Tofu with Eggplant	62
155.	Creamy Chicken Curry	62
156.	Garlic Bread Recipe	63
157.	Keto Cucumber Salad	63
158.	Cabbage Stir Fry	63
159.	Cauliflower Rice Bowl	64
160.	Golden Zucchini	64
161.	Tomato & Pepper Tapas	64
162.	Meaty Cream Cheese	64
163.	Wilted Spinach	65
164.	Cauliflower Soup	65
165.	Chicken and Broccoli	65
166.	Chorizo-Olive Sauce	66
167.	Chocolate Dessert	66
168.	Tantalizing Chocolate	66
169.	Perk You Up Porridge	67
170.	The Beastie Bacon Bagel	67
171.	Blueberry Whirl Mousse	67
172.	Strawberries smoothie	67
173.	Pumpkin Pie Custard	68
174.	Charismatic Crepes	68
175.	Coconut Curls	68
176.	Chicken Salad	68
177.	Grilled Ribeyes	69
178.	Beef & Asparagus	69
179.	Shrimp Scampi Spinach	69
180.	Almond Cheesecake	70
181.	Zesty Orange Ice Cream	70
182.	Chicken Parmesan	70
183.	Cajun Sirloin	71
184.	Sage-Rubbed Salmon	71
185.	Creamy Dijon Chicken	71
186.	Mom's Roast Chicken	72
187.	Cod and Asparagus Bake	72
188.	Parmesan Chicken	72
189.	Tuna & Cheese Oven Bake	73
190.	Tomato & Leek Bake	73
191.	Spicy Crab Pot Pie	73
192.	Garlic Bacon	73
193.	Spring roast chicken	74
194.	Shakshuka	74
195.	Hoisin Turkey Lettuce	74
196.	Keto Chicken Salad	75
197.	Kick-the-Boredom	75
198.	Oktoberfest Brats	75

199.	Chicken Breast	76
200.	Tuna Sushi Bites	76
201.	Mexican Salmon Fillets	76
202.	Masala frittata with avocado	77
203.	Coconut Chicken Soup	77
204.	Heavenly Gnocchi	77

KETO DINNER RECIPES 78

205.	Low Carb Sushi Roll	78
206.	Ketogenic Baked Eggs	78
207.	Pure Indulgence Peanut	79
208.	Cauliflower Rice	79
209.	Bulky Beef Pie	79
210.	Chicken Salad Stuffed	80
211.	Funky Fried Fish Cakes	80
212.	Greek bouyiourdi	80
213.	Chicken and Snap	81
214.	Low Carb Cauliflower	81
215.	Garlic Chicken	82
216.	Spicy Infused Shrimp	82
217.	Turkey Meatball	82
218.	Mighty Meaty Moussaka	83
219.	Creamy Keto Chicken	83
220.	Chicken Chasseur	83
221.	Spicy Salmon with Salsa	84
222.	Cashew Chicken	84
223.	Garlic Chicken Kebab	85
224.	Antipasto Meat Sticks	85
225.	Spicy Tuna Sushi Rolls	85
226.	Loaded Cauliflower	86
227.	Creamy Cauliflower	86
228.	Tasty Salted Turnip Fries	86
229.	Tantalizingly Tasty	87
230.	Eggs with Asparagus	87
231.	Greek Wedge Salad	87
232.	Perfect almond Cake	88
233.	Overnight Oats	88
234.	Strawberry Cashew Milk	88
235.	Continental pie	89
236.	Spicy Kick-Start	89
237.	Keto-Classic Cereal	89
238.	Mushroom baked	90
239.	Keto Pancakes	90
240.	Baked Egg	90
241.	Cobb Salad	90
242.	Shredded Fennel Salad	91
243.	Keto Coconut Macaroons	91
244.	Chicken Bacon Ranch	91
245.	Sandwich Lunchbox	92
246.	Keto-Buzz Blueberry	92
247.	Perfect Mozzarella	92
248.	What Waffle!	93
249.	Chile Relleno Casserole	93
250.	Keto Bacon Wrapped	93
251.	Roasted Chicken	94
252.	Crispy Keto Cauliflower	94

253.	Peanut Butter Cookies	95
254.	Keto Everything Bagel	95
l		95
255.	Bacon Cheeseburger Skillet	95
256.	Cheese & Tomato Salad	96
257.	Red Pepper and Basil	96
258.	Citrus Salmon	96
259.	Artichoke Chicken	96
260.	Zucchini Noodles	97
261.	Keto Tuna Salad	97
262.	Chicken & Goat Cheese	97
263.	Ginger Halibut with Brussels Sprouts	98
264.	Soy & butter salmon parcels	98
265.	Mexican Cabbage Roll	99
266.	Chicken Provolone	99
267.	Lemon-Pepper Tilapia	99
268.	Bountiful Bacon, Cheese	100
269.	Sensational Smoked	100
270.	Zucchini Noodles	100
271.	Tuna Burgers on a Bed	100
272.	Salmon & Creamy Spinach	101
273.	California Burger Wraps	101
274.	Chicken & pistachio salad	101
275.	Chicken Nicoise Salad	102
276.	Cauliflower & Ham Bake	102
277.	Moroccan Cauliflower	102
278.	Coconut Bed of Buttered	103
279.	Cheese Pancakes	103
280.	Butternut Squash	103

KETO VEGITARIAN RECIPES 104

281.	Broccoli Cheese Bites	104
282.	Keto Vegetable Bake	104
283.	Easy Cheesy Zucchini	105
284.	Low-Carb Spinach	105
285.	Keto Vegetable Soup	105
286.	Roasted Veggies	106
287.	Roasted Vegetable Salad	106
288.	Loaded Cauliflower	107
289.	Bacon Butter Roasted	107
290.	Keto Stir Fry	108
291.	Keto Tzatziki	108
292.	Cheese Pancakes	108
293.	Spinach and Cheese Pie	109
294.	Vegan Keto Breakfast	109
295.	Keto Butter Cauliflower	109
296.	Crispy Greek-style pie	110

SNACK AND DESSERTS RECIPES 110

297.	Fat Bombs	110
298.	Chocolate Chip Cookies	111
299.	Keto Cups	111
300.	Chip Cookie	111
301.	Keto Brownie Cookies	112
302.	Butter Fat Bombs	112
303.	No Bake Cookies	112

304.	Cheesecake Bites	113
305.	Chocolate Fat Bombs	113
306.	Smores Recipe	113
307.	Strawberry Cheesecake.......................	114
308.	Chocolate Chip	114
309.	Peanut Butter Chocolate Bars............	114
310.	Keto Chocolate Mousse	115
311.	Chocolate Crunch Bars	115
312.	Keto Lemon Bars	115
313.	Keto Chocolate	116
314.	Chocolate Fat Bombs	116
315.	Chocolate Fat Bombs	116
316.	Blueberry & pecan cookies	116

KETO SOUP RECIPES.. 117

317.	Broccoli & Pea Soup	117
318.	Green Vegetable Soup	117
319.	Keto Chicken Soup	117
320.	Keto Zuppa Toscana...........................	118
321.	Vegetable Soup Recipe	118
322.	Broccoli Cheddar Soup.......................	119
323.	Butter Mushroom Soup	119
324.	Asparagus Soup	119
325.	Chicken Coconut Soup	120
326.	Broccoli And Stilton Soup	120
327.	Keto Turkey Soup...............................	120
328.	Chilled green soup	121
329.	Vegetable Cabbage Soup	121
330.	Tomato Soup......................................	121
331.	Keto Tomato Soup	122

CONCLUSION 123

INTRODUCTION

"Since the 1960s, different variations of ketogenic diets have also become widely known as weight-loss methods," she says, and for some Americans, it's become their go-to way to control their weight. This might be a good option for some people, Leman says, because "the emphasis on 'whole foods' such as fish and seafood, low-carb vegetables, nuts, seeds and berries as the foundation of a keto diet is certainly healthier than the calorie-dense, nutrient-poor, refined, processed foods that form the foundation of the standard American diet."

In fact, Daryl Gioffre, celebrity nutritionist and author of "Get Off Your Acid," says that "anything is a good alternative to the standard American diet. The SAD diet is an extremely acidic diet that's pumped up with inflammatory foods, fats and sugars. It's literally wreaking havoc on peoples' health." The ketogenic diet — when done correctly — can be a great alternative, he says.

What is Keto Diet?

The ketogenic diet is just the opposite. It requires at least 70% of daily calories come from fat, only 5% to 10% from carbohydrates and about 25 percent from protein. On this diet, the body goes into a state of ketosis, where fat is burned for fuel instead of carbohydrate. The diet originated as a treatment for certain severe cases of epilepsy; for unknown reasons, ketosis reduces the occurrence and severity of these seizures.

Over the past few years, the keto diet has been promoted as a weight-loss tool for others.

And the anecdotal evidence suggests that, in the short term, it can result in quick and significant weight loss.

It may have other short-term benefits as well. A 2012 meta-analysis in the journal Obesity Reviews concluded that a low-carb diet did have "favorable effects" on major cardiovascular risk factors like body weight, blood pressure, cholesterol levels and blood sugar levels. However, "the effects on long-term health are unknown," it says.

One reason for that is because it is extremely difficult to maintain this eating style long term. Though it sounds like a carnivore's dream, eliminating practically all bread, cereal, pasta, sweets and other high-carb foods is, pardon the pun, no picnic.

How does the keto diet work?

The keto diet aims to force your body into using a different type of fuel. Instead of relying on sugar (glucose) that comes from carbohydrates (such as grains, legumes, vegetables, and fruits), the keto diet relies on ketone bodies, a type of fuel that the liver produces from stored fat.

Burning fat seems like an ideal way to lose pounds. But getting the liver to make ketone bodies is tricky:

- It requires that you deprive yourself of carbohydrates, fewer than 20 to 50 grams of carbs per day (keep in mind that a medium-sized banana has about 27 grams of carbs).
- It typically takes a few days to reach a state of ketosis.
- Eating too much protein can interfere with ketosis.

Benefits of keto diet?

There is a ton of hype Surrounding the ketogenic diet. Some researchers swear that it is the best diet for most people to be on, while others think it is just another fad diet. To some degree, both sides of the spectrum are right. There isn't one perfect diet for everyone or every condition, regardless of how many people "believe In It. The ketogenic diet is no exception to this rule. However, the ketogenic diet also has plenty of solid research backing up its benefit. It's better than most diets at helping people with:

- Epilepsy
- Parkinson's disease
- Fatty Liver Disease
- Type 2 Diabetes
- Type 1 Diabetes
- Cancer
- Chronic Inflammation
- High Blood Sugar
- Migraines
- High Blood Pressure Levels
- Ahheimer's disease
- Heart Disease

Even if you are not at risk from any of these conditions, the ketogenic diet can be helpful for you too. Some of the benefits that most people experience are:

- Better brain function
- A decrease in inflammation
- An increase in energy
- Improved body composition

What to Eat on a Keto Diet?

Keto emphasizes higher fat intake and little carb intake. This can make meal planning challenging since a large number of high carb foods are not considered keto-friendly - like grains, breads, starchy veggies, and fruits.

Additionally, carbs tend to be the bulk of most people's diets - meaning you have to find a keto alternative or change the way you think about meals in general. Some of the best staples for any keto diet should include healthy carb substitutes. Many veggies work great for this, like:

- Cauliflower rice
- Mashed cauliflower
- Portobello mushroom "buns"
- Spaghetti squash
- Zucchini noodles (or "zoodles")
- Lettuce wraps

Help keep your nutrition in check, have the bulk of your keto diet should consist of nutrient-rich low carb veggies, quality proteins, and healthy fats to ensure you are getting the right balance and overall good nutrition to keep you going.

Keto Food List

Here is a brief overview of what you should and shouldn't eat on the keto diet:

Do Not Eat
- Grains – wheat, corn, rice, cereal, etc.
- Sugar – honey, agave, maple syrup, etc.
- Fruit – apples, bananas, oranges, etc.
- Tubers – potato, yams, etc.

Do Eat
- Meats – fish, beef, lamb, poultry, eggs, etc.
- Low-carb vegetables – spinach, kale, broccoli, and other low carb veggies.

- High-fat dairy – hard cheeses, high fat cream, butter, etc.
- Nuts and seeds – macadamias, walnuts, sunflower seeds, etc.
- Avocado and berries – raspberries, blackberries, and other low glycemic impact berries
- Sweeteners – stevia, erythritol, monk fruit, and other low-carb sweeteners.
- Other fats – coconut oil, high-fat salad dressing, saturated fats, etc.

Healthy Fats

When following a high-fat, very-low-carb ketogenic (keto) diet, it's important to remember that not all fats are created equal.

Some sources of fat are better for you than others, and it's critical that you fill your plate with the most wholesome options to successfully reach your health goals.

Here are 14 healthy sources of fat to enjoy on the keto diet.

1. Avocados and avocado oil
2. Nuts
3. Nut and seed butters
4. Flax seeds
5. Hemp hearts
6. Chia seeds
7. Olives and cold-pressed olive oil
8. coconuts and unrefined coconut oil
9. Cacao nibs
10. Full-fat Greek yogurt
11. Whole eggs
12. Fatty fish
13. Butter
14. Cheese

What can I eat?

Cheese: Brie, cheddar, manchego, cream cheese – you name it. Finally, a diet that doesn't just allow cheese but encourages it, too.

Beef brisket: Enjoy this southern favorite with a side of homemade coleslaw.

Spinach: Avoid starchy root vegetables such as carrots or potatoes, and go for keto-friendly greens like spinach, broccoli, or kale. Use spinach for a salad, or blend a handful into your breakfast smoothie.

Bacon: Serve on the side with scrambled eggs (made out of pastured, organic whole eggs).

Yogurt: You may find sugar cravings don't disappear right away, so enjoy a bowl of yogurt or cottage cheese topped with berries to curb the cravings early on.

Cheeseburger: The keto diet favors fattier meats over lean meats, so don't be afraid to dig into a juicy burger – but skip the bun. Prepare with grass-fed ground beef and enjoy over a bed of lettuce.

Whole-fat milk: Add a splash in your morning coffee, but be careful before downing a glass of whole-fat milk with breakfast – while high in fat, it's also high in carbohydrates and should be consumed in moderation.

Chicken thighs: Baked chicken thighs are an easy dinner recipe to throw together. Though this meal needs at least 30 minutes in the oven, it requires less than five minutes to prepare.

Stevia: Steer clear of sugar and artificial sweeteners, and satisfy your sweet tooth with stevia instead.

What food can you eat on the Keto Diet?

Fatty animal protein: meat, bacon, eggs, poultry with skin and fish

Oils and natural fats: Olive, canola and palm oil, and cacao butter latte

Vegetables: Spinach, kale, lettuce, broccoli, and cucumbers

What food can't you eat on Keto Diet?

Alcohol: Not recommended during the ketosis phase

Sugar: This includes artificial sweeteners (use stevia instead).

What foods should you limit on Keto Diet?

Carbohydrates: Bread and pasta

Starchy root veggies: Potatoes, carrots, and turnips

How much does Keto Diet cost?

Meat – like grass-fed selections – and fresh veggies are more expensive than most processed or fast foods. What you spend on keto-friendly foods will vary with your choices of protein source and quality. You can select less-expensive, leaner cuts of meat and fatten them up with some oil. Buying less-exotic, in-season veggies will help keep you within budget.

Does Keto Diet have any health risks?

Keto could pose health risks, particularly for people with certain medical conditions. People with kidney or liver conditions should not attempt a keto diet.

Some experts caution that the diet can lead to muscle loss.

The keto diet isn't for everyone: Pregnant or nursing women, underweight people, or anyone with heart disease who hasn't first consulted a doctor should avoid the diet. Hormonal changes aren't always beneficial, as the diet can dramatically affect insulin and reproductive hormones. The keto diet for people with diabetes is controversial, and some dietitians advise against it. A person with diabetes, especially someone taking insulin, would require careful monitoring.

Keto diets take different paths, and your nutritional mileage may vary. You could incorporate healthy fats such as avocados and nuts as much as possible and focus on whole, unprocessed foods. In that case, the diet might have disease-preventing properties. On the other hand, if you choose to max out on the least-healthy sources of animal fats and protein like nitrate-packed processed meats, the diet could become part of the problem.

Recipe Notes

We wanted to make it as simple as possible for you to get in the kitchen and rustle up something special, so you will find each recipe laid out in an easy to follow format. Remember this diet is designed to rekindle your love of food not extinguish it with rules and regulations, so don't be afraid to experiment.

Use the ingredients as general guidelines and follow the instructions as best you can. You may not get everything the perfect first time, every time but that is what makes it yours! Keep at it for a full 30 days of eating and you will no doubt establish a few firm favourites that you can turn into your speciality dishes over time.

Each recipe ends with a breakdown of key nutritional information including the number of calories and amount of fats, carbohydrates and protein.

Again, this isn't to be obsessed over. Food is something to be enjoyed, so if you are going to keep a note of your intake levels then just make it a general estimate.

Why no pic? This cookbook is full of fun and flavour and doesn't take stuff too seriously. The food is entering your mouth, not a modelling contest, and we don't like to encourage unhealthy obsession about presentation. So just cook expert: tent, and enjoy.

Once you start loving what you are eating mealtimes will become something to look forward to. Take this as encouragement, go forth and cook to your heart's content!

28-Days Keto Diet Mealplan

Now, the moment you've been waiting for — the meal plan! In this chapter, you'll find a 28-day meal plan for the standard ketogenic diet, divided into four weeks. Every day you'll follow the plan to eat breakfast, lunch, and dinner, as well as a snack or dessert with a calorie range between 1,800 and 2,000.

One thing I want to mention before you get started is net carbs.

Many people who follow the ketogenic diet prefer to track net carbs rather than total carbs. To calculate net carbs, you simply take the total carb count of the meal and subtract the grams of fiber since fiber cannot be digested. Personally. I prefer to track total carbs like what I have mentioned in my first book, but I have included the grams of fiber and net carbs in these recipes, so you can choose which way to go.

personally, I prefer more buffer when it comes to the carb count, because I want to reduce the number of obstacles keeping me from ketosis. Many of my readers as well as friends have raised this point and you can be sure quite a few nights or afternoons were spent in heated debate! Okay, it wasn't that serious but suffice it to say that quite a bit of discussion went into this topic Therefore, I thought it might be better if I gave you a say in this net carb-total carb debate.

You get to choose whichever you prefer. In my personal opinion, when you are in the initial stages of trying to enter ketosis, keeping your total carb count in mind is probably one of the better practices you can adopt. A 20 to 50gram range of carbs would usually work to push the body into a ketogenic state.

After you have gotten keto adapted and the body gets used to burning fat for fuel, you on then start to bring net carbs into the equation. Keep in mind the calorie range for these meal plans — if you read my first book and calculated your own daily caloric needs, you may need to make some adjustments. If you're trying the ketogenic diet for the first time, however, it may be easiest to just follow the plan as is until you get the hang of it.

The first week of this 28-day meal plan is designed to be incredibly simple in terms of meal prep so want can focus on learning which foods to eat and which to avoid on the ketogenic diet — that's why you'll find more smoothies and soups here than in the following weeks. If you finish the first week and feel like you still need some time making the adjustment to keto, feel free to repeat it before moving on to week two. The meal plans also take into account left-overs and the yields of various recipes, so that you have minimal wage from your efforts in the kitchen. So, without further ado, let's take a look at the meal plans

28-Days Keto Diet Weight Loss Challenge

	First Week Meal Plan		
Day	**Breakfast**	**Lunch**	**Dinner**
Sunday	1.Bulletproof Coffee	103.Keto Guacamole	213.Chicken and Snap
Monday	14.Keto Oatmeal	104.Spicy Shrimp	219.Creamy Keto Chicken
Tuesday	2.Keto Butter Coffee	115.Keto chicken enchilada	242.Shredded Fennel Salad
Wednesday	3.Keto Boosted Coffee	107.Chewy Coconut Chunks	222.Cashew Chicken
Thursday	6.Coconut oil Coffee	111.Garlic Shrimp Zoodles	210.Chicken Salad Stuffed
Friday	14.Keto Oatmeal	115.Keto chicken enchilada	222.Cashew Chicken
Saturday	1.Bulletproof Coffee	103.Keto Guacamole	215.Garlic Chicken

28-Days Keto Diet Weight Loss Challenge

	Second Week Meal Plan		
Day	**Breakfast**	**Lunch**	**Dinner**
Sunday	1.Bulletproof Coffee	104.Spicy Shrimp	222.Cashew Chicken
Monday	14.Keto Oatmeal	107.Chewy Coconut Chunks	210.Chicken Salad Stuffed
Tuesday	2.Keto Butter Coffee	103.Keto Guacamole	215.Garlic Chicken
Wednesday	6.Coconut oil Coffee	107.Chewy Coconut Chunks	219.Creamy Keto Chicken
Thursday	14.Keto Oatmeal	111.Garlic Shrimp Zoodles	242.Shredded Fennel Salad
Friday	3.Keto Boosted Coffee	112.Garlic Gnocchi	222.Cashew Chicken
Saturday	1.Bulletproof Coffee	103.Keto Guacamole	213.Chicken and Snap

28-Days Keto Diet Weight Loss Challenge

Third Week Meal Plan

Day	Breakfast	Lunch	Dinner
Sunday	2.Keto Butter Coffee	103.Keto Guacamole	215.Garlic Chicken
Monday	6.Coconut oil Coffee	111.Garlic Shrimp Zoodles	242.Shredded Fennel Salad
Tuesday	3.Keto Boosted Coffee	104.Spicy Shrimp	219.Creamy Keto Chicken
Wednesday	1.Bulletproof Coffee	112.Garlic Gnocchi	222.Cashew Chicken
Thursday	3.Keto Boosted Coffee	107.Chewy Coconut Chunks	210.Chicken Salad Stuffed
Friday	14.Keto Oatmeal	107.Chewy Coconut Chunks	222.Cashew Chicken
Saturday	14.Keto Oatmeal	115.Keto chicken enchilada	213.Chicken and Snap

28-Days Keto Diet Weight Loss Challenge

Fourth Week Meal Plan			
Day	**Breakfast**	**Lunch**	**Dinner**
Sunday	1.Bulletproof Coffee	104.Spicy Shrimp	219.Creamy Keto Chicken
Monday	14.Keto Oatmeal	112.Garlic Gnocchi	242.Shredded Fennel Salad
Tuesday	6.Coconut oil Coffee	107.Chewy Coconut Chunks	222.Cashew Chicken
Wednesday	1.Bulletproof Coffee	107.Chewy Coconut Chunks	210.Chicken Salad Stuffed
Thursday	1.Bulletproof Coffee	111.Garlic Shrimp Zoodles	222.Cashew Chicken
Friday	3.Keto Boosted Coffee	103.Keto Guacamole	215.Garlic Chicken
Saturday	2.Keto Butter Coffee	115.Keto chicken enchilada	213.Chicken and Snap

Keto Breakfast Recipes

1. Bulletproof Coffee

Made for: Breakfast | **Prep Time:** 5 minutes | **Servings:** 01
Per Serving: Kcal: 320, Protein: 0g, Fat: 36g, Net Carb: 0g

INGREDIENTS

- ❖ 1 tbsp MCT Oil
- ❖ 2 tbsp Butter
- ❖ 12 oz Coffee

INSTRUCTIONS

1. Brew a cup of coffee using any brewing method you'd like.
2. Add butter, MCT oil, and coffee to a blender. Blend on high for 30 seconds. Enjoy.

2. Keto Butter Coffee

Made for: Breakfast | **Prep Time:** 5 minutes | **Servings:** 01
Per Serving: Kcal: 230, Protein: 0g, Fat: 25g, Net Carb: 0g

INGREDIENTS

- ❖ 1 cup (240 ml) of water
- ❖ 2 tbsp coffee
- ❖ 1 tbsp grass-fed butter
- ❖ 1 tbsp coconut oil

INSTRUCTIONS

1. Make a cup of coffee in your favourite way. We like to use Turkish Coffee Pot. We simply simmer ground coffee in water for about 5 minutes and then strain it into our cup. You can also use a Moka Pot, a French press, or a coffee machine!
2. Pour your brewed coffee into your blender (like a Nutribullet) and butter and coconut oil. Blend for about 10 seconds. You'll see it instantly become light and creamy!
3. Pour the butter coffee into a mug and enjoy! Add in any other ingredients you'd like in this step like cinnamon or whipped cream!

3. Keto Boosted Coffee

Made for: Breakfast | **Prep Time:** 3 minutes | **Servings:** 1

Per Serving: Kcal: 280, Protein: 1g, Fat: 31g, Net Carb: 1g

INGREDIENTS

- ❖ 2 cup (450 ml) freshly brewed hot coffee
- ❖ Two tablespoons grass-fed butter
- ❖ One scoop Perfect Keto MCT Powder
- ❖ One teaspoon Ceylon cinnamon

INSTRUCTIONS

1. Combine all of the ingredients in a blender.
2. Using an immersion blender or frother, blend on low bringing the speed up to high for 30 seconds or until frothy.
3. Serve, sip, and enjoy.

4. Keto Coffee Recipe

Made for: Breakfast | **Prep Time:** 7 minutes | **Servings:** 01
Per Serving: Kcal: 200, Protein: 1g, Fat: 22g, Net Carb: 0g

INGREDIENTS

- ❖ 12 oz freshly brewed coffee
- ❖ 1-2 tbsp Butter
- ❖ 1/4 tsp liquid stevia

INSTRUCTIONS

1. Add all ingredients to a blender jar and blend for 10 seconds.
2. Carefully remove the lid and pour into a coffee mug. See notes for other blending options.

5. Coconut oil Coffee

Made for: Breakfast | **Prep Time:** 5 minutes | **Servings:** 01
Per Serving: Kcal: 61, Protein: 0g, Fat: 6g, Net Carb: 0.1g

INGREDIENTS

- ❖ 1 cup (240 ml) coffee
- ❖ 1 1/2 tsp coconut oil
- ❖ 1/2 cup (120 ml) warm coconut milk ioptional
- ❖ 1/8 tsp cinnamon optional
- ❖ 1/8 tsp cayenne pepper optional
- ❖ Whole cloves for garnish
- ❖ Coconut cream for garnish
- ❖ Star anise for garnish

INSTRUCTIONS

1. Make a cup of coffee as you normally would and pour it into a blender.
2. Add the coconut oil to the blender and blend for 1-2 minutes until the mixture lightens in colour and becomes frothy.
3. Add any extras you'd like, including warm coconut milk, cinnamon, and or cayenne pepper, and give it a quick blend for 10-20 seconds.
4. Pour into a mug, top with coconut cream, and grind fresh cloves over the cream, if desired.
5. Garnish with star anise, and enjoy warm.

6. Cabbage Hash Browns

Made for: Breakfast | **Prep Time:** 25 minutes | **Servings:** 02
Per Serving: Kcal: 320, Protein: 28g, Fat: 60g, Net Carb: 4g

INGREDIENTS

❖ 2 large eggs
❖ 1/2 tsp. garlic powder
❖ 1/2 tsp. kosher salt
❖ Freshly ground black pepper
❖ 2 cup (140 g) shredded cabbage
❖ 1/4 small yellow onion, thinly sliced
❖ 1 tbsp. vegetable oil

INSTRUCTIONS

1. In a large bowl, whisk together eggs, garlic powder, and salt. Season with black pepper. Add cabbage and onion to egg mixture and toss to combine.
2. In a large skillet over medium-high heat, heat oil. Divide mixture into 4 patties in the pan and press with spatula to flatten. Cook until golden and tender, about 3 minutes per side.

7. Omelet-Stuffed Peppers

Made for: Breakfast | **Prep Time:** 40 minutes | **Servings:** 02
Per Serving: Kcal: 517, Protein: 20g, Fat: 48g, Net Carb: 7g

INGREDIENTS

❖ 2 bell peppers, halved and seeds removed

❖ 8 eggs, lightly beaten
❖ 1/4 cup (60 ml) milk
❖ 4 slices bacon, cooked and crumbled
❖ 1 cup (120 g) shredded cheddar
❖ 2 tbsp. finely chopped chives, plus more for garnish
❖ Kosher salt
❖ Freshly cracked black pepper

INSTRUCTIONS

1. Preheat oven to 400°. Place peppers cut side up in a large baking dish. Add a little water to the dish and bake peppers for 5 minutes.
2. Meanwhile, beat together eggs and milk. Stir in bacon, cheese, and chives and season with salt and pepper.
3. When peppers are done baking, pour egg mixture into peppers. Place back in the oven and bake 35 to 40 minutes more, until eggs are set. Garnish with more chives and serve.

8. Scrambled eggs with basil

Made for: Breakfast | Prep Time: 15 minutes | Servings: 02
Per Serving: Kcal: 625, Protein: 40g, Fat: 60g, Net Carb: 4g

INGREDIENTS

❖ 4 tbsp butter
❖ Four eggs
❖ 4 tbsp heavy whipping cream
❖ salt and ground black Pepper
❖ 4 oz/110 g shredded cheese
❖ 4 tbsp fresh basil

INSTRUCTIONS

1. Melt butter in a pan on low heat.
2. Add cracked eggs, cream, shredded cheese, and seasoning to a small bowl. Give it a light whisk and add to the pan.
3. Stir with a spatula from the edge towards the centre until the eggs are scrambled. If you prefer it soft and creamy, stir on lower heat until desired consistency.
4. Top with fresh basil.

9. Baked Eggs

Made for: Breakfast | **Prep Time:** 25 minutes | **Servings:** 2
Per Serving: Kcal: 338, Protein: 21g, Fat: 24g, Net Carb: 5g

INGREDIENTS

- ❖ 4 Eggs
- ❖ 4 Slices Bacon
- ❖ Salt and pepper to taste 1 Oz Cheddar
- ❖ 1 Small Onion (80g)

INSTRUCTIONS

1. Fry four slices of Bacon
2. Cut a small onion in half and fry
3. In a ramekin or equivalent ovenproof bowl, place onion and Bacon
4. Crack two eggs into each container, making sure to not break the yolk
5. Add salt and pepper
6. Add cheddar cheese
7. Bake at 350 degrees for 20 minutes or until eggs have set

10. Classic Bacon and eggs

Made for: Breakfast | **Prep Time:** 30 minutes | **Servings:** 4
Per Serving: Kcal: 270, Protein: 16g, Fat: 20g, Net Carb: 2g

INGREDIENTS

- ❖ Four eggs
- ❖ 2½ oz (70 g) bacon, in slices
- ❖ cherry tomatoes (optional)
- ❖ fresh parsley (optional

INSTRUCTIONS

1. Fry the Bacon in a pan on medium-high heat until crispy. Put aside on a plate. Leave the rendered fat in the pan.
2. Use the same pan to fry the eggs. Place it over medium heat and crack your eggs into the bacon grease. You can also crack them into a measuring cup and carefully pour into the pan to avoid splattering of hot grease.
3. Cook the eggs any way you like them. For sunny side up, leave the eggs to fry on one side and cover the pan with a lid to make sure they get cooked on top; for eggs

cooked over easy, flip the eggs over after a few minutes and cook for another minute. Cut the cherry tomatoes in half and fry them at the same time—salt and pepper to taste.

11. Mexican scrambled eggs

Made for: Breakfast | **Prep Time:** 25 minutes | **Servings:** 2
Per Serving: Kcal: 338, Protein: 21g, Fat: 24g, Net Carb: 5g

INGREDIENTS

- ❖ ½ oz (14g) butter
- ❖ ½ scallion, finely chopped
- ❖ One pickled jalapeño, finely chopped
- ❖ ½ tomato, finely chopped
- ❖ Three eggs
- ❖ 1½ oz (14 g) shredded cheese
- ❖ salt and pepper

INSTRUCTIONS

1. In a large frying pan, melt the butter over medium-high heat.
2. Add scallions, jalapeños, and tomatoes, and fry for 3-4 minutes.
3. Beat the eggs and pour ithem iinto the pan—scramble for 2 minutes. Add cheese and seasonings.

12. Keto English Muffins

Made for: Breakfast | **Prep Time:** 30 minutes | **Servings:** 1
Per Serving: Kcal: 340, Protein: 13g, Fat: 29g, Net Carb: 4g

INGREDIENTS

- ❖ 4 tablespoon Almond flour
- ❖ 1 Egg
- ❖ ½ teaspoon baking powder
- ❖ pinch salt
- ❖ 2 tablespoon Heavy cream/Double cream

INSTRUCTIONS

1. Place all of the ingredients into a small bowl, and whisk to combine completely.
2. Pour the batter into a well greased ramekin or mug, and microwave for 1 ½ minutes.
3. Let sit for several minutes, remove from the mug or ramekin, and cut in half.

4. Toast the muffin if desired before serving with your choice of toppings.

13. Seed & Nut Granola

Made for: Breakfast | **Prep Time:** 5 minutes | **Servings:** 1
Per Serving: Kcal: 400, Protein: 9.2g, Fat: 30g, Net Carb: 9g

INGREDIENTS

- ❖ Small handful of nuts (10 almonds, 3 Brazil nuts, 5 cashews)
- ❖ 2 Tablespoons (17 g) pumpkin seeds
- ❖ 1 Tablespoon (12 g) cacao nibs
- ❖ 1 Tablespoon (5 g) coconut flakes
- ❖ 1/4 cup (60 ml) unsweetened coconut

INSTRUCTIONS

1. Mix together all the dry ingredients. If you're making a large batch, then store leftovers in an airtight container.
2. Serve with coconut or almond milk.

14. Keto Oatmeal

Made for: Breakfast | **Prep Time:** 10 minutes | **Servings:** 01
Per Serving: Kcal: 381, Protein: 9g, Fat: 27g, Net Carb: 0.4g

INGREDIENTS

- ❖ Two tablespoons Golden Flaxseed Meal
- ❖ Two tablespoons Coconut Flour
- ❖ Two tablespoons Chia Seeds
- ❖ 1/2 cup (120 ml) Unsweetened Almond Milk
- ❖ Two tablespoons Heavy Cream
- ❖ 2-3 tablespoons Sugar-Free Maple Syrup
- ❖ One teaspoon Vanilla Essence

INSTRUCTIONS

1. Place the dry ingredients into a small saucepan and mix together.
2. Add the remaining ingredients.
3. Place the saucepan over medium heat and whisk the ingredients together for about 10 minutes until it has thickened and is warmed through.
4. Pour into a bowl and top with your favourite toppings - we recommend extra Sugar-Free Maple Syrup and chopped Pecans.

15. Low-Carb Baked Eggs

Made for: Breakfast | **Prep Time:** 15 minutes | **Servings:** 02
Per Serving: Kcal: 500, Protein: 30g, Fat: 34g, Net Carb: 2g

INGREDIENTS

- ❖ 6 ounces. Ground beef
- ❖ Four eggs
- ❖ 4 ounces. shredded cheese

INSTRUCTIONS

1. Preheat the oven to 400°F (200°C).
2. Arrange cooked ground-beef mixture in a small baking dish. Then make two holes with a spoon and crack the eggs into them.
3. Sprinkle shredded cheese on top.
4. Bake in the oven until the eggs are done, about 10-15 minutes.
5. Let cool for a while. The eggs and ground meat get very hot!

16. Mexican egg roll

Made for: Breakfast | **Prep Time:** 15 minutes | **Servings:** 02
Per Serving: Kcal: 132, Protein:10g, Fat: 9g, Net Carb: 1g

INGREDIENTS

- ❖ One large egg
- ❖ a little rapeseed oil for frying
- ❖ 2 tbsp tomato salsa
- ❖ about 1 tbsp fresh coriander

INSTRUCTIONS

1. Beat the egg with 1 tbsp water. Heat the oil in a medium nonstick pan. Add the egg and swirl around the base of the pan, as though you are making a pancake, and cook until set. There is no need to turn it.
2. Carefully tip the pancake onto a board, spread with the salsa, sprinkle with the coriander, then roll it up. It can be eaten warm or cold – you can keep it for two days in the fridge.

17. Keto Chia Pudding

Made for: Breakfast | **Prep Time:** 10 minutes | **Servings:** 01
Per Serving: Kcal: 155, Protein: 4g, Fat: 10g, Net Carb: 10g

INGREDIENTS

- ❖ 2 tablespoon chia seeds
- ❖ 1/2 cup (120 ml) almond milk or milk of choice
- ❖ 1 teaspoon honey or other sweetener, optional
- ❖ Strawberries or other fruits for topping

INSTRUCTIONS

1. Pour ingredients into a jar and mix well. Let settle for 2-3 minutes then mix again very well until you see no clumping.
2. Cover the jar and store in fridge overnight or for at least 2 hours.
3. When you're ready to eat it, top with your favorite fruit and enjoy cold!

18. Keto egg muffins

Made for: Breakfast | **Prep Time:** 25 minutes | **Servings:** 06
Per Serving: Kcal: 337, Protein: 24g, Fat: 26g, Net Carb: 2g

INGREDIENTS

- ❖ Two scallions, finely chopped
- ❖ 5 oz (140 g) chopped air-dried chorizo
- ❖ 12 eggs
- ❖ 2 tbsp red pesto or green pesto (optional)
- ❖ salt and Pepper
- ❖ 6 oz (170 g) shredded cheese

INSTRUCTIONS

1. Preheat the oven to 350°F (175°C).
2. Line a muffin tin with nonstick, insertable baking cups or grease a silicone muffin tin with butter.
3. Add scallions and chorizo to the bottom of the tin.
4. Whisk eggs together with pesto, salt, and pepper. Add the cheese and stir.
5. Pour the batter on top of the scallions and chorizo.
6. Bake for 15-20 minutes, depending on the size of the muffin tin.

19. Fried Tomatoes

Made for: Breakfast | **Prep Time:** 5 minutes | **Servings:** 01
Per Serving: Kcal: 320, Protein: 0g, Fat: 36g, Net Carb: 0g

INGREDIENTS

- ❖ 1 tsp rapeseed oil
- ❖ Three tomatoes halved
- ❖ Four large eggs
- ❖ 1 tbsp chopped parsley
- ❖ 1 tbsp chopped basil

INSTRUCTIONS

1. Heat the oil in a small nonstick frying pan, then cook the tomatoes cut-side down until starting to soften and colour. Meanwhile, beat the eggs with the herbs and plenty of freshly ground black pepper in a small bowl.
2. Scoop the tomatoes from the pan and put them on two serving plates. Pour the egg mixture into the pan and stir gently with a wooden spoon, so the egg that sets on the base of the pan moves to enable the uncooked egg to flow into space. Stop stirring when it's nearly cooked to allow it to put into an omelette. Cut into four and serve with the tomatoes.

20. Beef and Green Beans

Made for: Breakfast | **Prep Time:** 30 minutes | **Servings:** 02
Per Serving: Kcal: 698, Protein: 35g, Fat: 60g, Net Carb: 5g

INGREDIENTS

- ❖ 10 oz (280g) ground beef
- ❖ 9 oz (260g) fresh green beans
- ❖ 3½ oz (90g) butter
- ❖ salt and Pepper

INSTRUCTIONS

1. Rinse and trim the green beans.
2. Heat a generous dollop of butter in a frying pan where you can fit both the ground beef and the green beans.

3. Brown the ground beef on high heat until it's almost done. Add salt and pepper.
4. Lower the heat somewhat. Add more butter and fry the beans for 5 minutes in the same pan. Stir the ground beef now and then.
5. Season beans with salt and pepper. Serve with remaining butter and add mayonnaise or crème Fraiche if you need more fat for satiety.

21. Egg and Ham Rolls

Made for: Breakfast | **Prep Time:** 25 minutes | **Servings:** 04
Per Serving: Kcal: 158, Protein: 12g, Fat: 13g, Net Carb: 1g

INGREDIENTS

- ❖ 4 slices of ham
- ❖ One cucumber, sliced thin
- ❖ Four eggs whisked well
- ❖ 2 Tablespoons (30 ml) avocado oil, to cook with

INSTRUCTIONS

1. Add one teaspoon of avocado oil to a frying pan on low to medium heat and spread it around with a paper towel.
2. Add 1/4 cup of whisked eggs to the pan and roll it around to spread it thin.
3. Place a lid on top of the frying pan and let it cook until the base of the egg wrap is cooked (approx. 2-3 minutes). Carefully place on a plate and let cool.
4. Repeat in batches with the rest of the egg mixture to make egg wraps.
5. Create rolls with the egg wraps, slices of ham, and cucumber slices

22. Blueberry Smoothie

Made for: Breakfast | **Prep Time:** 5 minutes | **Servings:** 02
Per Serving: Kcal: 257, Protein: 10g, Fat: 20.5g, Net Carb: 5g

INGREDIENTS

- ❖ 1 large avocado
- ❖ 1/2 cup (10g) frozen blueberries
- ❖ 4 tsp flax seeds
- ❖ 2 tbsp collagen powder
- ❖ 1 1/2 cups (350 ml) of almond milk

INSTRUCTIONS

1. Put all the ingredients into a blender, and blend until smooth.

23. Cheese Omelette

Made for: Breakfast | **Prep Time:** 15 minutes | **Servings:** 01
Per Serving: Kcal: 511, Protein: 24g, Fat: 43g, Net Carb: 5g

INGREDIENTS

- ❖ 3 large mushrooms (sliced).
- ❖ 3 large eggs.
- ❖ 1 oz (30g) cheddar cheese (grated).
- ❖ 1 oz (25g) butter.
- ❖ ¼ onion (finely sliced).
- ❖ Pinch salt and pepper.

INSTRUCTIONS

1. In a bowl, whisk together the eggs, salt and pepper.
2. In a large frying pan, melt the butter and fry onions and mushrooms until tender.
3. Pour in the egg mixture so that it surrounds the onions and mushrooms.
4. As the sides begin to firm and it is still slightly runny in the middle, sprinkle on the cheese.
5. Continue cooking until egg mixture is completely formed and cooked through.

24. Spinach & Eggs

Made for: Breakfast | **Prep Time:** 15 minutes | **Servings:** 01
Per Serving: Kcal: 419, Protein: 13g, Fat: 40g, Net Carb: 1g

INGREDIENTS

- ❖ 2 large eggs.
- ❖ ½ cup (15g) baby spinach.
- ❖ 2 tbsp mayonnaise.
- ❖ 1 tbsp butter.
- ❖ Pinch salt and pepper.

INSTRUCTIONS

1. Melt butter in a large frying pan and crack

in the eggs.

2. As the eggs are frying, spoon over the melted butter from the pan until the yolk begins to have a white tint.
3. Place spinach on a plate with the mayonnaise, season with salt and pepper; place eggs next to spinach.

25.   Bacon & Egg

Made for: Breakfast | **Prep Time:** 15 minutes | **Servings:** 04
Per Serving: Kcal: 274, Protein: 17g, Fat: 24g, Net Carb: 1g

INGREDIENTS

❖ 8 large eggs.
❖ 5 oz (140g) bacon (slices).
❖ Handful of cherry tomatoes (halved).

INSTRUCTIONS

1. In a large frying pan, fry bacon rashers until crispy. Set aside, leaving bacon fat in the pan.
2. Crack the eggs into the frying pan and fry eggs to your preferred taste.
3. When eggs are nearly cooked, throw in the cherry tomatoes and fry until lightly browned.

26.   Egg Medley Muffins

Made for: Breakfast | **Prep Time:** 15 minutes | **Servings:** 02
Per Serving: Kcal: 320, Protein: 22g, Fat: 36g, Net Carb: 2g

INGREDIENTS

❖ 4 large eggs.
❖ 1/2 onion (finely chopped).
❖ 2 oz (60g) cheddar cheese (grated).
❖ 3 oz (85g) bacon (cooked and diced).
❖ Pinch salt and pepper.

INSTRUCTIONS

1. Preheat the oven at 175 degrees and grease a 12-hole muffin tray.
2. Equally, place onion and bacon to the bottom of each muffin tray hole.
3. In a large bowl, whisk the eggs, cheese, salt and pepper.

4. Pour the egg mixture into each hole; on top of the onions and bacon.
5. Bake for 20-25 minutes, until browned and firm to the touch.

27.   Cream Cheese Pancakes

Made for: Breakfast | **Prep Time:** 15 minutes | **Servings:** 01
Per Serving: Kcal: 346, Protein: 16g, Fat: 30g, Net Carb: 3g

INGREDIENTS

❖ 2 large eggs
❖ 2 oz cream cheese.
❖ 1 tsp granulated sugar substitute.
❖ ½ tsp ground cinnamon.

INSTRUCTIONS

1. Blend all ingredients until smooth. Allow to rest for 2 minutes.
2. Grease a large frying pan and pour in ¼ of the mixture.
3. Cook for 2 minutes until golden, flip and cook for an additional minute.
4. Repeat process until all mixture has gone.

28.   Cheese Egg Wrap

Made for: Breakfast | **Prep Time:** 15 minutes | **Servings:** 02
Per Serving: Kcal: 413, Protein: 24g, Fat: 33g, Net Carb: 4g

INGREDIENTS

❖ 3 large eggs.
❖ 5 oz/140g bacon (cooked and diced).
❖ 1 oz/30g cheddar cheese (grated).
❖ 1 tbsp tomato sauce (low carb).

INSTRUCTIONS

1. In a large bowl, whisk the eggs until smooth.
2. Heat a large non-stick frying pan and slowly pour in half of the egg mixture; ensuring it reaches the edge of the pan.
3. Cook until the edges begin to brown and crisp, flip and cook the other side for an additional 30-40 seconds. Repeat with remaining egg mixture.
4. Spread the cooked egg with tomato sauce and fill with cheese and bacon; roll into an egg wrap.

29.   Soldiers & Egg

Made for: Breakfast | **Prep Time:** 5 minutes | **Servings:** 01
Per Serving: Kcal: 270, Protein: 17g, Fat: 22g, Net Carb: 1g

INGREDIENTS

- ❖ 1 large egg.
- ❖ 2 oz (60g) cheddar cheese (cut in chunky wedges).

INSTRUCTIONS

1. Gently place the egg in a lidded saucepan of cold water, bring to the boil.
2. When the water is boiling excessively, turn off the heat and remove the pan away from the heat.
3. To create a soft and runny centre, leave the egg sitting in the hot water for 4 minutes.
4. Take the egg out of the water and crack off the top of the egg. Use the cheese sticks to dunk into the egg.

30.   Green Smoothie

Made for: Breakfast | **Prep Time:** 5 minutes | **Servings:** 01
Per Serving: Kcal: 380, Protein: 12g, Fat: 36g, Net Carb: 5g

INGREDIENTS

- ❖ 2 cups (60 g) spinach
- ❖ 1/3 cup (46 g) raw almonds
- ❖ 2 Brazil nuts
- ❖ 1 cup (240 ml) coconut milk
- ❖ 1 Tablespoon (10 g) psyllium seeds (or psyllium husks) or chia seeds

INSTRUCTIONS

1. Place the spinach, almonds, Brazil nuts, and coconut milk into the blender first.
2. Blend until pureed.
3. Add in the rest of the ingredients (greens powder, psyllium seeds) and blend well.

31.   Bacon Muffins

Made for: Breakfast | **Prep Time:** 25 minutes | **Servings:** 12
Per Serving: Kcal: 300, Protein: 11g, Fat: 28g, Net Carb: 4g

INGREDIENTS

- ❖ 3 cups (360g) almond flour
- ❖ 1 cup (100g) bacon bits
- ❖ 1/2 cup (120 ml) ghee
- ❖ 4 eggs, whisked
- ❖ 2 teaspoons (2g) lemon thyme
- ❖ 1 teaspoon (4g) baking soda

INSTRUCTIONS

1. Preheat oven to 350 F (175 C).
2. Melt the ghee in a mixing bowl.
3. Add in the rest of the ingredients except the bacon bits to the mixing bowl.
4. Mix everything together well.
5. Lastly, add in the bacon bits.
6. Line a muffin pan with muffin liners. Spoon the mixture into the muffin pan (to around 3/4 full).
7. Bake for 18-20 minutes until a toothpick comes out clean when you insert it into a muffin.

32.   Avocado Sandwich

Made for: Breakfast | **Prep Time:** 15 minutes | **Servings:** 01
Per Serving: Kcal: 544, Protein: 23g, Fat: 46g, Net Carb: 11g

INGREDIENTS

- ❖ 6 slices bacon.
- ❖ 2 avocados.
- ❖ 2 small onions (diced).
- ❖ 2 tbsp lime juice.
- ❖ 2 tbsp garlic powder.
- ❖ Cooking spray.

INSTRUCTIONS

1. Preheat the oven at 180 degrees.
2. Spray a baking tray with cooking spray, cook the bacon 20-25 minutes until crispy.
3. Remove seeds from avocados; in a large bowl mash avocado flesh with a fork.
4. Add onions, garlic and lime juice; mash until well combined.
5. Allow the crispy bacon to cool and place one slice on a plate; top with 2 tbsp of avocado guacamole. Place another bacon slice on top and add another 2 tbsp of guacamole and

top with bacon. Repeat to make another sandwich.

33. Breakfast Porridge

Made for: Breakfast | **Prep Time:** 5 minutes | **Servings:** 02
Per Serving: Kcal: 430, Protein: 8g, Fat: 40g, Net Carb: 6g

INGREDIENTS

- ❖ 1/2 cup (60 g) almonds, ground using a food processor or blender
- ❖ 3/4 cup (180 ml) coconut milk
- ❖ 1 teaspoon (2 g) cinnamon powder
- ❖ Dash of nutmeg
- ❖ Dash of cloves

INSTRUCTIONS

1. Heat the coconut milk in a small saucepan on medium heat until it forms a liquid.
2. Add in the ground almonds and sweetener and stir to mix in.
3. Keep stirring for approximately 5 minutes (it'll start to thicken a bit more).
4. Add in the spices (have a taste to check whether you want more sweetener or spices) and serve hot.

34. Scrambled Eggs

Made for: Breakfast | **Prep Time:** 10 minutes | **Servings:** 01
Per Serving: Kcal: 318, Protein: 17g, Fat: 26g, Net Carb: 1.8g

INGREDIENTS

- ❖ 1 tbsp of unsalted butter
- ❖ 3 Large Eggs
- ❖ Coarse salt & freshly ground pepper

INSTRUCTIONS

1. Beat together the eggs using a fork.
2. In a medium nonstick pan, melt the butter over low heat.
3. Add the egg mixture.
4. Use a heatproof flexible spatula to pull the eggs gently to the center of the skillet. *Let the liquid parts run out under the perimeter*.

5. Cook, keep moving eggs around using the spatula for 2-3 minutes, just until the eggs are set.
6. Add salt and pepper to season. Serve hot.

35. Avocado Coconut Milk

Made for: Breakfast | **Prep Time:** 5 minutes | **Servings:** 01
Per Serving: Kcal: 437, Protein: 5g, Fat: 43g, Net Carb: 10g

INGREDIENTS

- ❖ ½ avocado
- ❖ ½ cup (120 g) Unsweetened Coconut Milk
- ❖ 5 drops stevia
- ❖ 5 Ice Cubes

INSTRUCTIONS

1. Add all the ingredients to the blender. Blend until smooth.

36. Fried Avocados

Made for: Breakfast | **Prep Time:** 5 minutes | **Servings:** 02
Per Serving: Kcal: 200, Protein: 2g, Fat: 10g, Net Carb: 2g

INGREDIENTS

- ❖ 1 ripe avocado (not too soft), cut into slices
- ❖ 1 Tablespoon (15 ml) coconut oil
- ❖ 1 Tablespoon (15 ml) lemon juice
- ❖ Salt to taste

INSTRUCTIONS

1. Add coconut oil to a frying pan. Place the avocado slices into the oil gently.
2. Fry the avocado slices (turning gently) so that all sides are slightly browned.
3. Sprinkle the lemon juice and salt over the slices and serve warm

37. Veggie breakfast bakes

Made for: Breakfast | **Prep Time:** 40 minutes | **Servings:** 04
Per Serving: Kcal: 127, Protein: 09g, Fat: 08g, Net Carb: 05g

INGREDIENTS

- ❖ 4 large field mushrooms
- ❖ 8 tomatoes , halved

- ❖ 1 garlic clove , thinly sliced
- ❖ 2 tsp olive oil
- ❖ 200g bag spinach
- ❖ 4 eggs

INSTRUCTIONS

1. Heat oven to 200C/180C fan/gas 6. Put the mushrooms and tomatoes into 4 ovenproof dishes. Divide garlic between the dishes, drizzle over the oil and some seasoning, then bake for 10 mins.
2. Meanwhile, put the spinach into a large colander, then pour over a kettle of boiling water to wilt it. Squeeze out any excess water, then add the spinach to the dishes. Make a little gap between the vegetables and crack an egg into each dish. Return to the oven and cook for a further 8-10 mins or until the egg is cooked to your liking

38. Cauliflower Hash

Made for: Breakfast | **Prep Time:** 15 minutes | **Servings:** 02
Per Serving: Kcal: 189, Protein: 15g, Fat: 18g, Net Carb: 4g

INGREDIENTS

- ❖ 2 large eggs.
- ❖ 12 oz cauliflower rice (frozen).
- ❖ Olive oil for frying.
- ❖ ½ cup (80g) parmesan (grated).
- ❖ ½ tsp salt.
- ❖ ¼ tsp black pepper.
- ❖ ⅛ tsp paprika.

INSTRUCTIONS

1. Microwave the cauliflower rice and allow to soften.
2. Mix all ingredients, except the eggs, together with the rice until well combined.
3. When the mixture is thoroughly combined, stir in the eggs and mix well.
4. Heat olive oil in a large frying pan and scoop 1 heaped tbsp of mixture into the pan. Fry for 2 minutes on each side until crispy and golden brown.
5. Repeat process until all mixture has gone.

39. Butter Breakfast Balls

Prep Time: 60 minutes | **Servings:** 15 balls
Per Ball: Kcal: 173, Protein: 8g, Fat: 15g, Net Carb: 6g

INGREDIENTS

- ❖ 2 cups peanut butter (smooth).
- ❖ ¾ cup (95 g) coconut flour.
- ❖ ½ cup (170 g) erythritol or monk fruit sweetened maple syrup.

INSTRUCTIONS

1. Line a large baking tray with greaseproof paper.
2. In a large bowl, mix all ingredients together until a thick batter is formed.
3. Mould the batter into small balls and place on the baking tray.
4. Refrigerate 40-60 minutes until firm.

40. Keto deviled eggs

Made for: Breakfast | **Prep Time:** 15 minutes | **Servings:** 02
Per Serving: Kcal: 170, Protein: 08g, Fat: 16g, Net Carb: 1g

INGREDIENTS

- ❖ ½ tsp tabasco
- ❖ 2 tbsp mayonnaise
- ❖ ½ pinch herbal salt
- ❖ 4 cooked and peeled shrimp
- ❖ fresh dill

INSTRUCTIONS

1. Start by boiling the eggs by placing them in a pot and covering them with water. Place the pot over medium heat and bring to a light boil.
2. Boil for 8-10 minutes to make sure the eggs are hardboiled.
3. Remove the eggs from the pot and place in an ice bath for a few minutes before peeling.
4. Split the eggs in half and scoop out the yolks.
5. Place the egg whites on a plate.
6. Mash the yolks with a fork and add tabasco, herbal salt and homemade mayonnaise.

7. Add the mixture, using two spoons, to the egg whites and top with a shrimp on each, or a piece of smoked salmon.
8. Decorate with dill.

41.   Tuna & Spinach Mix

Made for: Breakfast | **Prep Time:** 15 minutes | **Servings:** 02
Per Serving: Kcal: 952, Protein: 53g, Fat: 80g, Net Carb: 3g

INGREDIENTS

- ❖ 4 large eggs.
- ❖ 10 oz tinned tuna (in olive oil).
- ❖ ½ cup (230 g) mayonnaise.
- ❖ 1 avocado (sliced).
- ❖ 1 onion (finely diced).
- ❖ Salt and pepper (to season).

INSTRUCTIONS

1. Bring a large pan of water to the boil and lower in the eggs. Cook for 8 minutes.
2. In a bowl, mix together tuna, mayonnaise, onion, salt and pepper.
3. Chop the hard boiled eggs into halves and place on a plate with avocado slices and spinach.
4. Place the tuna mixture on top of spinach.

42.   Keto mushroom omelet

Made for: Breakfast | **Prep Time:** 20 minutes | **Servings:** 02
Per Serving: Kcal: 230, Protein: 16g, Fat: 21g, Net Carb: 2g

INGREDIENTS

- ❖ 6 eggs
- ❖ 2 oz (56 g) butter, for frying
- ❖ 2 oz (55 g) shredded cheese
- ❖ ½ yellow onion, chopped
- ❖ 8 large mushrooms, sliced
- ❖ salt and pepper

INSTRUCTIONS

1. Crack the eggs into a mixing bowl with a pinch of salt and pepper.
   Whisk the eggs with a fork until smooth and frothy.

2. Melt the butter in a frying pan, over medium heat. Add the mushrooms and onion to the pan, stirring until tender, and then pour in the egg mixture, surrounding the veggies.
3. When the omelet begins to cook and get firm, but still has a little raw egg on top, sprinkle cheese over the egg.
4. Using a spatula, carefully ease around the edges of the omelet, and then fold it over in half. When it starts to turn golden brown underneath, remove the pan from the heat and slide the omelet on to a plate.

43.   Almond Butter Choco

Made for: Breakfast | **Prep Time:** 5 minutes | **Servings:** 01
Per Serving: Kcal: 190, Protein: 4g, Fat: 5g, Net Carb: 3g

INGREDIENTS

- ❖ 1 cup (240 ml) coconut milk or almond milk
- ❖ 2 Tablespoons (10 g) unsweetened cacao powder (or 1 scoop CoBionic Indulgence for added collagen)
- ❖ 1 Tablespoon (16 g) almond butter
- ❖ 1 teaspoon (5 ml) vanilla extract

INSTRUCTIONS

1. Place all the ingredients into a blender and blend well.

44.   Fried Halloumi Cheese

Made for: Breakfast | **Prep Time:** 15 minutes | **Servings:** 02
Per Serving: Kcal: 830, Protein: 36g, Fat: 74g, Net Carb: 7g

INGREDIENTS

- ❖ 10 oz. mushrooms
- ❖ 10 oz. halloumi cheese
- ❖ 3 oz. butter
- ❖ 10 green olives
- ❖ salt and pepper

INSTRUCTIONS

1. Rinse and trim the mushrooms, and cut or slice.

2. Heat up a hearty dollp of butter in a frying pan where you can fit both halloumi cheese and mushrooms.
3. Fry the mushrooms on medium heat for 3-5 minutes until they are golden brown. Season with salt and pepper.
4. If necessary, add more butter and fry the halloumi for a couple of minutes on each side. Stir the mushrooms every now and then. Lower the heat towards the end. Serve with olives.

45. Tomato baked eggs

Made for: Breakfast | **Prep Time:** 50 minutes | **Servings:** 04
Per Serving: Kcal: 204, Protein: 09g, Fat: 16g, Net Carb: 4g

INGREDIENTS

- ❖ 900g (6 cup) ripe vine tomatoes
- ❖ 3 garlic cloves
- ❖ 3 tbsp olive oil
- ❖ 4 large free range eggs
- ❖ 2 tbsp chopped parsley or chives

INSTRUCTIONS

1. Preheat the oven to fan 180C/ conventional 200C/gas 6. Cut the tomatoes into quarters or thick wedges, depending on their size, then spread them over a fairly shallow 1.5 litre ovenproof dish. Peel the garlic, slice thinly and sprinkle over the tomatoes. Drizzle with the olive oil, season well with salt and pepper and stir everything together until the tomatoes are glistening.
2. Slide the dish into the oven and bake for 40 minutes until the tomatoes have softened and are tinged with brown.
3. Make four gaps among the tomatoes, break an egg into each gap and cover the dish with a sheet of foil. Return it to the oven for 5-10 minutes until the eggs are set to your liking. Scatter over the herbs and serve piping hot with thick slices of toast or warm ciabatta and a green salad on the side.

46. Chives Egg Muffins

Made for: Breakfast | **Prep Time:** 35 minutes | **Servings:** 04
Per Serving: Kcal: 240, Protein: 12g, Fat: 22g, Net Carb: 3g

INGREDIENTS

- ❖ 6 eggs
- ❖ 1 cup kale, finely chopped
- ❖ 1/4 cup (17 g) chives, finely chopped
- ❖ 1/2 cup (120 ml) almond or coconut milk
- ❖ Salt and pepper to taste

INSTRUCTIONS

1. Preheat the oven to 350 F (175 C).
2. Whisk the eggs and add in the chopped kale and chives. Also add in the almond/coconut milk, salt, and pepper. Mix well.
3. Grease 8 muffin cups with coconut oil or line each cup with a prosciutto slice.
4. Divide the egg mixture between the 8 muffin cups. Fill only 2/3 of each cup as the mixture rises when it's baking.
5. Bake in oven for 30 minutes.
6. Let cool a few minutes and then lift out carefully with a fork. Note that the muffins will sink a bit.

47. Filling Veg Soup

Made for: Breakfast | **Prep Time:** 25 minutes | **Servings:** 4
Per Serving: Kcal: 85, Protein: 9g, Fat: 13g, Net Carb: 3g

INGREDIENTS

- ❖ 4 cups (800ml) vegetable broth.
- ❖ 2 tins tomatoes
- ❖ 2 bell peppers
- ❖ 4 cloves garlic (crushed).
- ❖ 1 cauliflower (cut into florets).
- ❖ 2 tbsp olive oil.
- ❖ 1 tbsp Italian seasoning.

INSTRUCTIONS

1. Heat olive oil in a large saucepan.
2. Saute onions and bell peppers for 10 minutes until tender and lightly browned; stir in garlic and cook for an additional minute.
3. Add the broth, cauliflower, tomatoes and

Italian seasoning; bring to the boil. Cover, reduce heat and simmer for 20-25 minutes until the veg is tender.

48. Turkey Wrap

Made for: Breakfast | **Prep Time:** 25 minutes | **Servings:** 01
Per Serving: Kcal: 360, Protein: 20g, Fat: 30g, Net Carb: 3g

INGREDIENTS

- ❖ 2 slices of turkey breast (use more if the slices break easily)
- ❖ 2 romaine lettuce leaves (or 2 slices of avocado)
- ❖ 2 slices of bacon
- ❖ 2 eggs
- ❖ 1 Tablespoon (15 ml) coconut oil to cook in

INSTRUCTIONS

1. Cook the 2 slices of bacon to the crispness you like.
2. Scramble the 2 eggs in the coconut oil (or bacon fat).
3. Make 2 wraps by placing half the scrambled eggs, 1 slice of bacon, and 1 romaine lettuce leaf on each slice of turkey breast.

49. Oven-Baked Brie Cheese

Made for: Breakfast | **Prep Time:** 15 minutes | **Servings:** 04
Per Serving: Kcal: 342, Protein: 15g, Fat: 31g, Net Carb: 1g

INGREDIENTS

- ❖ 9 oz. Brie cheese or Camembert cheese
- ❖ 1 garlic clove, minced
- ❖ 1 tbsp fresh rosemary, coarsely chopped
- ❖ 2 oz. pecans or walnuts, coarsely chopped
- ❖ 1 tbsp (15 ml) olive oil
- ❖ salt and pepper

INSTRUCTIONS

1. Preheat the oven to 400°F (200°C).
2. Place the cheese on a sheet pan lined with parchment paper or in a small non-stick baking dish.
3. In a small bowl, mix the garlic, herb and nuts together with the olive oil. Add salt and

pepper to taste.
4. Place the nut mixture on the cheese and bake for 10 minutes or until cheese is warm and soft and nuts are toasted. Serve warm or lukewarm.

50. Keto cheese omelet

Made for: Breakfast | **Prep Time:** 15 minutes | **Servings:** 02
Per Serving: Kcal: 897, Protein: 40g, Fat: 80g, Net Carb: 4g

INGREDIENTS

- ❖ 3 oz. butter
- ❖ 6 eggs
- ❖ 7 oz. shredded cheddar cheese
- ❖ salt and pepper to taste

INSTRUCTIONS

1. Whisk the eggs until smooth and slightly frothy. Blend in half of the shredded cheddar. Salt and pepper to taste.
2. Melt the butter in a hot frying pan. Pour in the egg mixture and let it set for a few minutes.
3. Lower the heat and continue to cook until the egg mixture is almost cooked through. Add the remaining shredded cheese. Fold and serve immediately.

51. Keto smoked salmon

Made for: Breakfast | **Prep Time:** 10 minutes | **Servings:** 02
Per Serving: Kcal: 1016, Protein: 33g, Fat: 97g, Net Carb: 1g

INGREDIENTS

- ❖ 12 oz. smoked salmon
- ❖ 1 cup/230g mayonnaise
- ❖ 2 cups/30g baby spinach
- ❖ 1 tbsp/15 ml olive oil
- ❖ ½ lime (optional)
- ❖ salt and pepper

INSTRUCTIONS

1. Put salmon, spinach, a wedge of lime, and a hearty dollop of mayonnaise on a plate.
2. Drizzle olive oil over the spinach and season with salt and pepper.

52. Keto Breakfast Burrito

Made for: Breakfast | **Prep Time:** 6 minutes | **Servings:** 01
Per Serving: Kcal: 330, Protein: 11g, Fat: 30g, Net Carb: 1g

INGREDIENTS

- ❖ 1 tbsp (14 g) butter
- ❖ 2 cggs medium
- ❖ 2 tbsp cream full fat/ 15g Double cream
- ❖ choice of herbs or spices
- ❖ salt/pepper to taste

INSTRUCTIONS

1. In a small bowl, whisk the eggs, cream and chosen herbs and spices.
2. Melt the butter in the frying pan then pour in the burrito egg mixture.
3. Swirl the frying pan until the burrito mixture is evenly spread and thin as shown in the cooking video.
4. Place a lid over the burrito and leave to cook for 2 minutes.
5. Gently lift the burrito from the frying pan with a clean spatula onto a plate.
6. Add your favourite fillings then roll up and enjoy.

53. Baked Broccoli Bites

Made for: Breakfast | **Prep Time:** 35 minutes | **Servings:** 4
Per Serving: Kcal: 175, Protein: 11g, Fat: 8g, Net Carb: g

INGREDIENTS

- ❖ 300 g (4 cup) Broccoli, chopped
- ❖ 3 slices Wholemeal bread, blended into bread crumbs
- ❖ ½ Onion, finely diced
- ❖ 60 g (1/4 cup) Mature Cheese
- ❖ 2 Eggs, beaten
- ❖ 1 teaspoon Garlic powder
- ❖ 1 teaspoon Dried oregano
- ❖ 1 pinch Sea salt and black pepper

INSTRUCTIONS

1. Add the broccoli to a pan of boiling water and simmer for 3 minutes. Drain and then add to a large bowl and mash until very fine.

2. Add the rest of the ingredients to the bowl and mix well.
3. Take out 1 tablespoon at a time and roll in to a small sausage and repeat until you have 20.
4. Place on a lined or oiled baking sheet and cook in a preheated oven at 200°C/400°F for 25 minutes until they start to crisp up. Serve with your favourite dip.

54. Keto breakfast sandwich

Made for: Breakfast | **Prep Time:** 35 minutes | **Servings:** 01
Per Serving: Kcal: 600, Protein: 22g, Fat: 56g, Net Carb: 4g

INGREDIENTS

- ❖ 2 sausage patties
- ❖ 1 egg
- ❖ 1 tbsp cream cheese
- ❖ 2 tbsp sharp cheddar
- ❖ 1/4 medium avocado, sliced
- ❖ 1/4-1/2 tsp sriracha (to taste)
- ❖ Salt, pepper to taste

INSTRUCTIONS

1. In skillet over medium heat, cook sausages per package instructions and set aside
2. In small bowl place cream cheese and sharp cheddar. Microwave for 20-30 seconds until melted
3. Mix cheese with sriracha, set aside
4. Mix egg with seasoning and make small omelette
5. Fill omelette with cheese sriracha mixture and assemble sandwich

55. Pancake Recipe

Made for: Breakfast | **Prep Time:** 15 minutes | **Servings:** 02
Per Serving: Kcal: 257, Protein: 18g, Fat: 18g, Net Carb: 5g

INGREDIENTS

- ❖ 3 (3) Eggs
- ❖ 1/2 cup (105 g) cottage cheese
- ❖ 1/3 cup (37.33 g) Superfine Almond Flour
- ❖ 1/4 cup (62.5 g) Unsweetened Almond Milk
- ❖ 2 tablespoons (2 tablespoons) Truvia
- ❖ Vanilla extract

- ❖ 1 teaspoon (1 teaspoon) Baking Powder
- ❖ Cooking Oil Spray

INSTRUCTIONS

1. Place ingredients in a blender jar in the order listed.
   Blend until you have a smooth, liquid batter.
2. Heat a nonstick saucepan on medium-high heat. Spray with oil or butter.
3. Place 2 tablespoons of batter at a time to make small, dollar pancakes. This is a very liquid, delicate batter so do not try to make big pancakes with this one as they will not flip over as easily.
4. Cook each pancake until the top of the pancake has made small bubbles and the bubbles have disappeared, about 1-2 minutes.
5. Using a spatula, gently loosen the pancake, and then flip over.
6. Make the rest of the pancakes in this manner and serve hot.

56.   Keto Breakfast

Made for: Breakfast | **Prep Time:** 25 minutes | **Servings:** 4
Per Serving: Kcal: 126, Protein: 3g, Fat: 10g, Net Carb: 5g

INGREDIENTS

- ❖ 1 large turnip peeled and diced
- ❖ 1/4 onion diced
- ❖ 1 cup (90g) brussel sprouts halved
- ❖ 3 slices bacon
- ❖ 1 tablespoon olive oil
- ❖ 1/2 teaspoon paprika
- ❖ 1/2 teaspoon garlic powder
- ❖ 1/2 teaspoon salt
- ❖ 1/2 teaspoon black pepper
- ❖ 1/4 cup (110g) red bell pepper diced
- ❖ 1 Tbsp Parsley for garnish

INSTRUCTIONS

1. Add the oil to a large skillet over medium high heat.
2. Add in the turnips and spices.
3. Cook 5-7 minutes stirring occasionally.

4. Add in the onion and brussel sprouts and cook 3 minutes until they starts to soften.
5. Chop the bacon into small pieces and add to the skillet, along with red bell pepper. (Add the bacon in with the turnips if you like it crispy)
6. Continue to cook another 5-7 minutes until the bacon is cooked.
7. Garnish with parsley before serving.

57.   Cheese & Bacon

Made for: Breakfast | **Prep Time:** 25 minutes | **Servings:** 08
Per Serving: Kcal: 207, Protein: 10g, Fat: 18g, Net Carb: 3g

INGREDIENTS

- ❖ 1 cauliflower head (florets).
- ❖ 8 oz (225 g) bacon (in strips).
- ❖ 3 oz (85 g) butter.
- ❖ ⅔ cup (60 g) parmesan (grated).
- ❖ ⅓ cup (38 g) mozzarella (grated).
- ❖ ½ tsp black pepper.

INSTRUCTIONS

1. Preheat the oven at 200 degrees.
2. Bring a large pan of water to the boil, add cauliflower and cook for 7-8 minutes until tender.
3. Drain the water and add butter and pepper. Blend until cauliflower is a smooth puree.
4. In a frying pan, fry bacon until crispy. Add half of the bacon and all juice to the puree; along with half of the parmesan.
5. Stir well and pour into an ovenproof dish.
6. Sprinkle over the remaining bacon, parmesan and mozzarella.
7. Bake for 20-25 minutes until the cheese is melted and golden.

58.   Buttered Cabbage

Made for: Breakfast | **Prep Time:** 5 minutes | **Servings:** 01
Per Serving: Kcal: 380, Protein: 4g, Fat: 43g, Net Carb: 3g

INGREDIENTS

- ❖ 5 oz cabbage (cut in long strips).
- ❖ 2 oz butter.
- ❖ 2 bacon slices.

INSTRUCTIONS

1. In a large frying pan, melt half of the butter and fry the bacon until crispy.
2. Add the remaining butter and stir in the cabbage; cook until cabbage begins to change colour.

59. Bacon & Spinach Bake

Made for: Breakfast | **Prep Time:** 35 minutes | **Servings:** 04
Per Serving: Kcal: 660, Protein: 28g, Fat: 61g, Net Carb: 4g

INGREDIENTS

- ❖ 8 large eggs.
- ❖ 8 oz (225g) fresh spinach.
- ❖ 1 cup (230g) thick cream or double cream.
- ❖ 5 oz (140g) bacon (diced).
- ❖ 5 oz cheddar cheese (grated).
- ❖ 2 tbsp butter.

INSTRUCTIONS

1. Preheat the oven at 175 degrees.
2. In a large frying pan, melt the butter and fry the bacon until crispy. Add in the spinach and fry until wilted. Set aside.
3. In a large bowl, whisk together the eggs and cream.
4. Pour the egg mixture into an ovenproof dish; add bacon and spinach and top with cheese.
5. Bake for 25-30 minutes until completely set and golden brown.

60. Cauliflower Medley

Made for: Breakfast | **Prep Time:** 5 minutes | **Servings:** 02
Per Serving: Kcal: 650, Protein: 31g, Fat: 59g, Net Carb: 5g

INGREDIENTS

- ❖ 10 oz beef (minced, frozen & defrosted).
- ❖ 8 oz cauliflower (florets).
- ❖ 3 oz butter.
- ❖ 1 tsp paprika.
- ❖ 1 tsp black pepper.
- ❖ ½ tsp salt.

INSTRUCTIONS

1. Melt half of the butter in a large frying pan and fry the beef until almost cooked through.
2. Lower the heat; add the remaining butter, season with paprika, salt and pepper. Stir in the cauliflower and fry for 5-6 minutes until tender.

61. Olive Feast

Made for: Breakfast | **Prep Time:** 10 minutes | **Servings:** 02
Per Serving: Kcal: 849, Protein: 33g, Fat: 77g, Net Carb: 9g

INGREDIENTS

- ❖ 10 oz halloumi (cut into slices).
- ❖ 1 aubergine (cut into bite size pieces).
- ❖ 3 oz butter.
- ❖ 12 olives (pitted).
- ❖ 1 tsp paprika.
- ❖ 1 tsp chilli flakes.

INSTRUCTIONS

1. Melt the butter in a large frying pan.
2. Place the aubergine chunks and olives in one half and halloumi in the other.
3. Season with paprika and chilli; cook for 8-10 minutes, turning occasionally to ensure halloumi is golden brown on both sides and aubergine is cooked through.

62. Lime Pancakes

Prep Time: 10 minutes | **Servings:** 10 Pancakes
Per Pancakes: Kcal: 27, Protein: 9g, Fat: 28g, Net Carb: 4g

INGREDIENTS

- ❖ 4 eggs.
- ❖ 2 cups/225g almond flour.
- ❖ ¼ cup/75g water.
- ❖ 8 tbsp butter (melted).
- ❖ 2 tbsp swerve.
- ❖ 1 tbsp coconut oil.
- ❖ 1 tsp baking powder.
- ❖ 1 lime zest.
- ❖ 1 lemon zest.

INSTRUCTIONS

1. Place all ingredients in a blender and blend until well combined.
2. Allow to rest for 10-15 minutes.
3. In a frying pan heat a little oil, pour in ⅓ cup of batter mixture.
4. Cook for 2-3 minutes on each side until golden brown.
5. Repeat the process until all of the batter has gone.

63. Keto Crepes Recipe

Made for: Breakfast | **Prep Time:** 15 minutes | **Servings:** 04
Per Serving: Kcal: 690, Protein: 14g, Fat: 70g, Net Carb: 4g

INGREDIENTS

- ❖ 8 large eggs.
- ❖ 2 cups (480g) thick whipping cream.
- ❖ ½ cup (125ml) water (room temperature).
- ❖ 3 oz butter.
- ❖ 2 tbsp psyllium husk (powder).

INSTRUCTIONS

1. In a large bowl, whisk together eggs, cream and water. Gradually mix in the psyllium husk until a smooth batter is formed. Allow to rest for 20 minutes.
2. Use a little butter and ½ cup of batter mixture for one pancake.
3. When the top of the pancake is lightly browned and almost dry, flip and cook the other side.
4. Repeat until all batter has gone.

64. Wraps with Avocado

Made for: Breakfast | **Prep Time:** 15 minutes | **Servings:** 02
Per Serving: Kcal: 459, Protein: 27g, Fat: 40g, Net Carb: 4g

INGREDIENTS

- ❖ 2 Almost Zero Carb Wraps
- ❖ 3 slices bacon cooked
- ❖ 2 large eggs
- ❖ 1/2 cup (55g) grated cheddar cheese
- ❖ 1/2 avocado sliced
- ❖ 1/4 cup (65g) salsa
- ❖ salt and pepper to taste

INSTRUCTIONS

1. Cook the bacon in the pan until crisp. Remove, cut in half and set aside. Pour out all but 2 teaspoons of bacon fat. Slice the avocado.
2. In a small bowl, beat the eggs and half of the cheddar cheese cheese with a fork. Cook the scrambled eggs to your liking and remove from the pan. Season with salt and pepper.
3. Place the wraps into the hot pan over medium heat (I had to overlap mine just a bit in the middle). Divide the scrambled eggs and place them on 1/2 of each wrap, not going past the middle. Add the avocado, bacon and remaining cheese. Add 1 tablespoon of water to the pan and cover quickly with a lid. Leave covered for 1-2 minutes or until the cheese has melted and the bottom of the wraps have browned a bit. Serve with salsa.

65. Peanut Butter Cookies

Prep Time: 20 minutes | **Servings:** 06 Cookies
Per Cookies: Kcal: 200, Protein: 10g, Fat: 18g, Net Carb: 3.5g

INGREDIENTS

- ❖ ½ cup (125 g) creamy peanut butter
- ❖ 4.oz. cream cheese
- ❖ ½ cup (45 g) Sukrin gold or golden monkfruit sweetener
- ❖ ½ teaspoon baking soda
- ❖ 1 small egg

INSTRUCTIONS

1. Gather all of your ingredients for the peanut butter cookies in one place.
2. Preheat oven to 350F and line a cookie sheet with baking paper.
3. In a mixing bowl, combine creamy peanut butter, cream cheese, sweetener, baking soda, and the egg. Also, add vanilla extract if you're using.
4. Once the ingredients are combines, the mixture should look like this.

5. Next place the mixed batter into a fridge for 20 minutes.
6. Once the time is up, separate the batter into 6 scoops and place onto the baking sheet.
7. Bake the ketogenic peanut butter cookies for 12-14 minutes or until golden.
8. The cookies will be soft once removed from the oven, but they will firm up after cooling for a few minutes.

66. Bacon Cheddar Egg Cups

Made for: Breakfast | **Prep Time:** 25 minutes | **Cups:** 6
Per Cup: Kcal: 190, Protein: 12g, Fat: 15g, Net Carb: 1g

INGREDIENTS

- ❖ 6 medium eggs
- ❖ 1 cup (130g) grated turnip or kohlrabi
- ❖ 6 slices bacon, cooked (180 g/ 6.4 oz)
- ❖ 1/4 cup (57 g) grated cheddar cheese
- ❖ pinch of salt and black pepper, to taste

INSTRUCTIONS

1. Place the bacon in a hot pan and cook for a few minutes. Turn and cook for a few more minutes. The bacon should be cooked but still soft (not too crispy).
2. Preheat oven to 190 °C/ 375 °F (conventional), or 170 °C/ 340 °F (fan assisted). Divide the grated turnip between 6 silicone muffin molds. Place a strip of bacon into the mold around the edges.
3. Keto Bacon Cheddar Egg Cups
4. Place a tablespoon of cheese into the mold

   then crack an egg into each mold.
5. Keto Bacon Cheddar Egg Cups
6. Transfer to oven for 20-25 minutes or until set. Eat warm or cold. Store in the fridge for up to 4 days.

67. Broccoli and Cheddar

Made for: Breakfast | **Prep Time:** 25 minutes | **Servings:** 12
Per Serving: Kcal: 94, Protein: 6g, Fat: 6g, Net Carb: 1g

INGREDIENTS

- ❖ 1/2 tsp dried thyme
- ❖ 1/2 tsp garlic powder
- ❖ 1 1/2 cups (276 g) broccoli steamed and chopped (or frozen and thawed)
- ❖ 2/3 cup (75 g) grated cheddar cheese plus more for topping

INSTRUCTIONS

1. Whisk in garlic powder and thyme until combined. Stir in broccoli and cheddar. Divide evenly into muffin tins1 filling each about 2/3 full.
2. Sprinkle with more cheddar if desired. Bake in preheated oven for 12-15 minutes, or until set.

68. Strawberry Fat Bombs

Made for: Breakfast | **Prep Time:** 30 minutes | **Servings:** 09
Per Serving: Kcal: 330, Protein: 0g, Fat: 31g, Net Carb: 2g

INGREDIENTS

- ❖ 15 fresh medium sized Strawberries
- ❖ 7-ounce cream cheese, softened
- ❖ 1 teaspoon stevia
- ❖ 3 tablespoon butter, softened at room temperature
- ❖ 1 teaspoon vanilla extract

INSTRUCTIONS

1. In a blender blitz the fresh strawberries until they break up and puree consistency forms.
2. In a bowl mix cream cheese, vanilla extract, stevia and butter together.
3. When well mixed, add in the purred strawberries and mix them until fully incorporated and combined.
4. Place the bowl in fridge for about 30 minutes.
5. Scoop out some of the mixture and serve or eat yourself.
6. Enjoy.

69. Buffalo Chicken

Made for: Breakfast | **Prep Time:** 25 minutes | **Servings:** 2
Per Serving: Kcal: 94, Protein: 6g, Fat: 6g, Net Carb: 1g

INGREDIENTS

- ❖ 1/3 cup (94g) Buffalo Sauce I used Frank's
- ❖ 1/3 cup (32g) chopped green onions
- ❖ 1 cup (150g) chopped cooked or rotisserie chicken

INSTRUCTIONS

1. Whisk in garlic powder and buffalo sauce until combined. Stir in green onions. Divide evenly into muffin cups filling each about 2/3 full.
2. Use a spoon to evenly distribute chicken into muffin cups (about 2-3 tablespoons each). Bake in preheated oven for 12-15 minutes, or until set. Serve with a drizzle of buffalo sauce if desired.

70.   Simple keto breakfast

Made for: Breakfast | **Prep Time:** 10 minutes | **Servings:** 01
Per Serving: Kcal: 424, Protein: 13g, Fat: 41g, Net Carb: 1g

INGREDIENTS

- ❖ 2 eggs
- ❖ 1 tbsp butter
- ❖ 2 tbsp mayonnaise
- ❖ 1 oz. (1 cup) baby spinach
- ❖ salt and ground black pepper to taste
- ❖ 1 cup/230ml coffee or tea

INSTRUCTIONS

1. Heat butter in a frying pan over medium heat.
2. Crack your eggs straight into the pan. For eggs sunny side up – leave the eggs to fry on one side. For eggs cooked over easy – flip the eggs over after a few minutes and cook for another minute. For harder yolks, just leave cooking for a few more minutes. Season with salt and pepper.
3. Serve with baby spinach, a dollop of mayonnaise, and a cup of freshly brewed black coffee or a cup of tea.

71.   Keto Breakfast Cake

Made for: Breakfast | **Prep Time:** 20 minutes | **Servings:** 04
Per Serving: Kcal: 430, Protein: 12g, Fat: 39g, Net Carb: 8g

INGREDIENTS

- ❖ 4 tablespoons butter
- ❖ 6 eggs
- ❖ 4 oz. softened cream cheese
- ❖ 1/4 cup (50 g) granular erythritol
- ❖ 1/2 cup (120 g) heavy cream/Double Cream
- ❖ 1/4 cup (28 g) coconut flour
- ❖ 2 teaspoons almond extract

INSTRUCTIONS

1. Heat your oven to 425°F.
2. Place the butter in a cast iron skillet (or other oven-proof skillet) and transfer to the oven.
3. Meanwhile, mix the remaining ingredients together in a mixing bowl to make the batter.
4. Carefully with oven mitts or a pot holder, remove the skillet from the oven when the butter is melted and pour batter into skillet. Make sure the batter covers the bottom of the skillet completely.
5. Bake for 15-18 minutes or until it gets bubbly and golden brown.
6. Top with confectioner erythritol, slivered almonds, and sugar-free syrup before serving.

72.   Ham and Cheddar

Made for: Breakfast | **Prep Time:** 15 minutes | **Servings:** 04
Per Serving: Kcal: 528, Protein: 22g, Fat: 36g, Net Carb: 9g

INGREDIENTS

- ❖ 8 slices white bread
- ❖ A little butter for spreading
- ❖ 4 slices of ham
- ❖ 50g (1/4 cup) Cheddar, sliced
- ❖ 5 large eggs
- ❖ salt and freshly ground black pepper
- ❖ 3tbsp oil for frying

INSTRUCTIONS

1. Spread the slices of bread on one side with a little butter, then make four ham and cheese

sandwiches in the normal way. Beat the eggs with salt and freshly ground black pepper. Dip two sandwiches in the egg, letting it soak in a little.
2. Heat half the oil in a large non-stick frying pan, then add the sandwiches to the hot frying pan. Cook for 3 mins until the base is golden, then carefully turn over with a spatula. Cook for a further 3 mins or until golden on the base.
3. Transfer to a plate and keep warm. Repeat to make the remaining sandwiches in the same way. Serve cut in half with a few cherry tomatoes if liked.

73. Keto Breakfast Bake

Made for: Breakfast | **Prep Time**: 35 minutes | **Servings**: 12
Per Serving: Kcal: 265, Protein: 16g, Fat: 21g, Net Carb: 1g

INGREDIENTS

- ❖ 1/2 green pepper, chopped
- ❖ 1 pound (450 g) Black Forest or smoked Deli ham chopped
- ❖ 2 tablespoon butter
- ❖ 7 eggs
- ❖ 3/4 cup (180 ml) heavy whipping cream/Double cream
- ❖ 2 cups (256 g) cheddar cheese
- ❖ 1/2 teaspoon salt
- ❖ 1/4 teaspoon pepper

INSTRUCTIONS

1. Preheat oven to 350 degrees.
2. In a skillet, saute green peppers and chopped deli ham until the peppers begin to soften, and the ham is nice and browned.
3. Grease a 9 X 13 casserole dish.
4. Place the ham and peppers in the casserole dish.
5. In a bowl, combine the beaten eggs, heavy whipping cream, salt, and pepper and whisk until all the ingredients are thoroughly combined.
6. Pour egg mixture over the ham and green peppers then sprinkle cheese on top. Use a fork to stir ingredients around to make sure

that all of the ham is covered with the egg and cheese mixture.
7. Bake for 20-23 minutes, depending on how done you like your eggs.

74. Bacon Egg and Cheese

Prep Time: 35 minutes | **Bites**: 24
Per Bites: Kcal: 75, Protein: 3g, Fat: 6g, Net Carb: 1g

INGREDIENTS

- ❖ 4 large eggs
- ❖ 2 ounces cream cheese, softened
- ❖ 1 cup chopped cooked bacon (5-6 thick slices)
- ❖ 1 1/4 cups (78 g) shredded cheese (I like to do a combination of cheddar and pepper jack)
- ❖ 1/3 cup (112 g) coconut flour OR almond flour
- ❖ 1/2 teaspoon baking powder

INSTRUCTIONS

1. Preheat oven to 350 degrees F.
2. In a medium size mixing bowl, combine all of the ingredients. Make sure to break up the cream cheese as you stir.
3. Allow the mixture to sit for 10 minutes for the flour to absorb some of the moisture. DO NOT SKIP THIS STEP!
4. Spray a regular mini muffin pan or use a silicone muffin pan (my recommendation) and fill each cup about 3/4 full.
5. Bake 15-18 minutes until golden brown and cooked through.

75. Keto Kimchi

Made for: Breakfast | **Prep Time**: 25 minutes | **Servings**: 12
Per Serving: Kcal: 23, Protein: 1g, Fat: 1g, Net Carb: 2g

INGREDIENTS

- ❖ 1 Chinese (or Napa) cabbage (1.5 lb or 700 g), washed and quartered lengthwise
- ❖ 1/3 cup (75 g) salt, to wilt the cabbage

For the kimchi sauce:
- ❖ 1 Tablespoon fresh ginger
- ❖ 12 cloves of garlic (approx. 1 head of garlic), peeled

- 1/2 small red onion, peeled
- 1 small chili pepper, seeds removed
- 1 Tablespoon crushed red chili pepper
- 1/4 cup (60 ml) hot sauce, or to taste
- 1 Tablespoon (15 g) salt

INSTRUCTIONS

1. Sprinkle salt liberally on the quartered cabbage. Place into a container for 2-3 hours so the water flows out of the cabbage. Pour out the water.
2. Wash the cabbage again to remove the excess salt. Wring the cabbage gently with your hands to remove excess water.
3. To make the kimchi sauce, blend the sauce ingredients.
4. Use your hands to massage the kimchi sauce over the cabbage.
5. Marinate for 1 day at room temperature.
6. Keep in fridge and consume within 2 weeks. Chop the cabbage into small pieces when serving.

76.   Breakfast Fat Bombs

Made for: Breakfast | **Prep Time:** 5 minutes | **Servings:** 01
Per Serving: Kcal: 360, Protein: 12g, Fat: 36g, Net Carb: 2g

INGREDIENTS

- 4 hardboiled eggs chopped
- 8 ounces cream cheese
- 2 tablespoons minced green onion
- 1 lb bacon cooked and crumbled

INSTRUCTIONS

1. In a medium bowl mix together the egg, cream cheese, and green onion. Roll into 8 balls. Place the balls in the freezer for 10 minutes to set just a bit.
2. Place the crumbled bacon on a plate and roll the balls in the bacon pressing the bacon slightly into the ball. Store in an airtight container in the refrigerator for up to 4 days.

77.   Breakfast Cookies

Made for: Breakfast | **Prep Time:** 35 minutes | **Servings:** 04
Per Serving: Kcal: 250, Protein: 14g, Fat: 16g, Net Carb: 3g

INGREDIENTS

- 1/2 cup (56 g) flaked coconut
- 1/2 cup (45 g) sliced almonds
- 1/2 cup (100 g) Swerve Brown
- 1/3 cup collagen peptides
- 1/2 cup (120 g) almond butter slightly melted
- 1 large egg
- 1 tsp maple extract
- 1/2 tsp vanilla extract

INSTRUCTIONS

1. Preheat the oven to 350F and line a large rimmed baking sheet with a silicone liner.
2. In a food processor, combine the coconut and almonds, and grind until they resemble oat flakes. Add the sweetener and collagen, and pulse a few more times to combine.
3. Transfer to a large bowl and stir in the almond butter, egg, and extracts until well combined. Use about 2 tablespoons for each cookie and roll into balls.
4. Place on the prepared baking sheet and press down to about 1/2 inch thick. Bake 15 to 20 minutes, until golden and firm to the touch. Remove and let cool on the pan. Do note: the cookies may release a lot of grease during baking but this will reabsorb as they cool.

78.   Breakfast Casserole

Made for: Breakfast | **Prep Time:** 65 minutes | **Servings:** 02
Per Serving: Kcal: 210, Protein: 13g, Fat: 15g, Net Carb: 4g

INGREDIENTS

- ½ cup (70 g) onion
- 1 Tbsp garlic, minced
- 1 lb breakfast sausage
- 12 eggs
- ½ cup (125 ml) milk of choice
- 2 tsp mustard powder
- 1 tsp oregano
- ¼ tsp salt
- pepper, to taste
- 1½ cups (42 g) broccoli florets

- 1 zucchini/ Courgette, diced
- 1 red bell pepper, diced

INSTRUCTIONS

1. Preheat oven to 375°F (190°C).
2. In a skillet over medium heat, add a drizzle of oil and sauté onion and garlic.
3. Once transparent, add sausage and cook until browned, 7-10 minutes.
4. Add to a 13×9-inch casserole or baking dish and set aside.
5. In a large bowl, whisk together eggs, milk of choice, and seasonings. Stir in chopped veggies.
6. Pour mixture over sausage. (Feel free to sprinkle on some shredded cheese, if desired!)
7. Bake until firm and cooked through, 30-40 minutes.
8. Allow to cool slightly before slicing into squares, serving, and enjoying!
9. Store leftovers in the fridge for up to 5 days, and reheat individual portions in the microwave.

79.   Egg Breakfast Wraps

Made for: Breakfast | **Prep Time:** 15 minutes | **Servings:** 02
Per Serving: Kcal: 470, Protein: 27g, Fat: 38g, Net Carb: 4g

INGREDIENTS

- 2 Almost Zero Carb Wraps
- 3 slices bacon cooked
- 2 large eggs
- 1/2 cup (56 g) grated cheddar cheese
- 1/2 avocado sliced
- 1/4 cup (65 g) salsa
- salt and pepper to taste

INSTRUCTIONS

1. Cook the bacon in the pan until crisp. Remove, cut in half and set aside. Pour out all but 2 teaspoons of bacon fat. Slice the avocado.
2. In a small bowl, beat the eggs and half of the cheddar cheese cheese with a fork. Cook the

scrambled eggs to your liking and remove from the pan. Season with salt and pepper.
3. Place the wraps into the hot pan over medium heat (I had to overlap mine just a bit in the middle). Divide the scrambled eggs and place them on 1/2 of each wrap, not going past the middle. Add the avocado, bacon and remaining cheese. Add 1 tablespoon of water to the pan and cover quickly with a lid. Leave covered for 1-2 minutes or until the cheese has melted and the bottom of the wraps have browned a bit. Serve with salsa.

80.   Breakfast Sandwich

Made for: Breakfast | **Prep Time:** 35 minutes | **Servings:** 04
Per Serving: Kcal: 500, Protein: 22g, Fat: 29g, Net Carb: 7g

INGREDIENTS

- 3 eggs
- ½ cup (110 g) of cream cheese
- 1 pinch of salt
- ½ tablespoon of baking powder (About 3 grams approx.
- 4 slices of ham
- 4 slices of cheddar cheese
- 8 thin slices of tomato (the equivalent of a small tomato)
- 4 slices of cucumber
- 2 slices of avocado
- 2 lettuce leaves
- Dressings to taste: pepper, oregano, vinegar, salt.

INSTRUCTIONS

1. Preheat the oven to 150 ° C.
2. Separate the white and yolk of the eggs, beat the egg whites until stiff, when you get firm peaks, add the salt. Reserve this mixture.
3. Mix the yolks with the cream cheese and add the yeast. Add this dough to the whites little by little stirring in an enveloping way so as not to lose the fluffiness of the whites in its point. With a ladle, place 6 large spoons separated from each other in a tray lined with baking paper.

4. Bake for 25 to 30 minutes until brown, and allow to cool; then, unmold carefully.
5. You can fill these sandwiches to your liking; I chose to fill them with ham, cheddar cheese, fresh lettuce, tomato, avocado slices and cucumber.
6. In addition, you can season with a pinch of oregano, pepper and a teaspoon of olive oil.

81. Breakfast Scramble

Made for: Breakfast | **Prep Time:** 15 minutes | **Servings:** 01
Per Serving: Kcal: 320, Protein: 7g, Fat: 36g, Net Carb: 2g

INGREDIENTS

- ❖ 2 eggs
- ❖ Kosher salt and pepper to taste
- ❖ 1 tablespoon olive oil or butter
- ❖ 1 medium avocado, diced
- ❖ Hot sauce (optional)

INSTRUCTIONS

1. Dice the avocado and set aside.
2. In a medium bowl, whisk together eggs with salt and pepper until light and fluffy.
3. Heat butter or olive oil in a small skillet over medium heat. Pour in the egg mixture. Once the eggs start to cook, reduce heat to medium-low and scramble them as they cook, stirring constantly.
4. Add in the diced avocados while the eggs are cooked halfway through and scramble together.
5. Cook for another minute and serve warm with hot sauce, if desired.

82. Low-Carb Keto

Made for: Breakfast | **Prep Time:** 5 minutes | **Servings:** 01
Per Serving: Kcal: 450, Protein: 21g, Fat: 43g, Net Carb: 5g

INGREDIENTS

- ❖ 2 eggs
- ❖ 1 tbsp cream (skip if paleo)
- ❖ 1 tsp butter
- ❖ 3 slices bacon (50g)
- ❖ 1 large crimini mushroom (40g)
- ❖ 4 broccoli sticks (60g)
- ❖ 1/4 avocado (40g)
- ❖ pinch salt
- ❖ pinch black pepper

INSTRUCTIONS

1. Add some water to a pot and heat.
2. Add the broccoli sticks to the boiling water and cook for 2-3 minutes.
3. Add the bacon slices to a frying pan and cook on both sides until nice and crispy. Don't discard of the oil.
4. Slice the shiitake mushroom and avocado.
5. Take the broccoli out of the water and add them to the bacon grease along with the mushroom slices.
6. Fry in the bacon grease until nice and tender.
7. In a small bowl, whisk the eggs and cream together.
   *For this step you can either fry the eggs inside the grease or fry them in some ghee.
8. Scramble the eggs until desired thickness.
9. Add your fried eggs, avocado, broccoli, bacon and mushrooms to a plate. Sprinkle the salt & pepper over.

83. Keto Breakfast Pockets

Made for: Breakfast | **Prep Time:** 35 minutes | **Servings:** 08
Per Serving: Kcal: 250, Protein: 6g, Fat: 20g, Net Carb: 5g

INGREDIENTS

- ❖ 8 oz mozzarella cheese shredded or cubed
- ❖ 2 oz cream cheese
- ❖ ⅔ cup (74g) almond flour
- ❖ ⅓ cup (38g) coconut flour
- ❖ 1 egg
- ❖ 2 tsp baking powder
- ❖ 1 tsp salt
- ❖ 2 eggs scrambled
- ❖ 4 oz Canadian bacon
- ❖ ½ cup (14g) shredded cheddar cheese

INSTRUCTIONS

1. Preheat oven to 350.

2. Put mozzarella cheese and the cream cheese in a microwave-safe bowl. Microwave one minute. Stir. Microwave 30 seconds. Stir. At this point, all the cheese should be melted. Microwave 30 more seconds (it should look like cheese fondue at this point).
3. Put the melted cheese and the other dough ingredients into a food processor and pulse until a uniform dough forms. (Alternatively, you can mix by hand but make sure to knead the dough thoroughly).
4. Divide the dough into 8 pieces. Press each into a 6-inch circle on a piece of parchment paper on a baking sheet. It helps to wet your hands. Divide the filling between each circle of dough. Fold in the edges and crimp to seal. Place back on the parchment seam side down.
5. Bake for 20-25 minutes until golden brown.

84. Breakfast Bowl

Made for: Breakfast | **Prep Time:** 5 minutes | **Servings:** 01
Per Serving: Kcal: 402, Protein: 24g, Fat: 36g, Net Carb: 3g

INGREDIENTS

- ❖ 2 large eggs
- ❖ 3 slices bacon
- ❖ 3 cups collard greens
- ❖ 1/4 tsp black pepper
- ❖ 1/2 tsp Pink Himalayan Salt
- ❖ 1/4 tsp garlic powder
- ❖ 1/2 tbsp ghee

INSTRUCTIONS

1. Heat a large skillet to medium-high heat and slice up the bacon into pieces. Add the bacon to the hot pan and allow to cook down.
2. Once the bacon is cooked to your liking add in the collard greens and season with garlic powder, salt and pepper. Cook the collards down to your liking and then transfer bacon and collards to a bowl.
3. Add the ghee to the hot pan and crack in the eggs. Let them fry up until the white is fully cooked through and season them with salt

and pepper. Once the eggs are cooked add them to your bowl and enjoy!

85. Keto Tasty Casserole

Made for: Breakfast | **Prep Time:** 35 minutes | **Servings:** 08
Per Serving: Kcal: 309, Protein: 21g, Fat: 26g, Net Carb: 3g

INGREDIENTS

- ❖ 10 whole eggs
- ❖ 2 cups diced ham
- ❖ 2 cups (56g) shredded cheddar cheese divided
- ❖ ⅓ cup (80ml) heavy cream/double cream
- ❖ ½ cup (75g) red bell pepper seeded, ribs removed and chopped
- ❖ ¼ cup (38g) onions minced
- ❖ ½ teaspoon salt
- ❖ ¼ teaspoon pepper

INSTRUCTIONS

1. Preheat oven to 350F.
2. Add in the eggs, heavy cream, salt and pepper into a large mixing bowl and mix using a hand mixer for about 2 minutes, until combined and fluffy.
3. Stir in the ham, peppers, onions and a little less than half of the shredded cheese.
4. Pour the mixture into a 9" x 13" casserole baking dish that's been sprayed with nonstick spray. Top with the remaining cheese and bake for 25-30 minutes or until the eggs have set and the cheese is golden and bubbly. Mine took exactly 30 minutes.

86. Bacon Cheddar Keto

Made for: Breakfast | **Prep Time:** 30 minutes | **Servings:** 06
Per Serving: Kcal: 252, Protein: 13g, Fat: 21g, Net Carb: 3g

INGREDIENTS

- ❖ Non-stick cooking spray
- ❖ 2 tbsp extra virgin olive oil
- ❖ 3 cups broccoli florets
- ❖ 3 tbsp water
- ❖ 1 cup (28g) shredded sharp cheddar or Colby Jack
- ❖ 6 slices bacon cooked and crumbled

- ❖ 4 large eggs
- ❖ 1/3 cup (80ml) heavy whipping cream/double cream
- ❖ 1/2 tsp onion powder
- ❖ 1/2 tsp garlic powder
- ❖ 1/4 tsp dried thyme
- ❖ 1/2 tsp dried oregano
- ❖ Salt and pepper to taste
- ❖ Fresh parsley optional garnish

INSTRUCTIONS

1. Preheat oven to 350 F and spray an 8" x 8" casserole dish with non-stick cooking spray. Set aside.
2. Heat the olive oil in a large nonstick sauté pan over medium heat. Add the broccoli and water and cook for 2-3 minutes, or just until the broccoli softens slightly and turns bright green.
3. Remove from heat and drain thoroughly. Transfer the broccoli to prepared casserole dish and spread into a uniform layer. Top with shredded cheese and crumbled bacon and side aside.
4. Whisk the eggs with the heavy cream, onion powder, garlic powder, thyme, and oregano. Season with salt and pepper, as desired. Pour the egg mixture over the broccoli, cheese, and bacon and bake for 17-23 minutes, or until the casserole is set and lightly golden brown on top.
5. Remove from oven and let cool for 10 minutes before slicing. If desired, sprinkle with fresh parsley.

87. Chia Seeds Bread

Prep Time: 25 minutes | Breads: 12
Per Breads: Kcal: 148, Protein: 5g, Fat: 12g, Net Carb: 2g

INGREDIENTS

- ❖ 4 eggs
- ❖ 1/4 cup (60g) almond milk or water
- ❖ 1/2 teaspoon salt
- ❖ 1 cup almond flour
- ❖ 1/4 cup (60g) melted butter
- ❖ 2 teaspoons baking soda
- ❖ 1/2 cup (85g) chia seeds (this is optional)

INSTRUCTIONS

1. Add everything into a bowl and stir well until you got an even mass.
2. Pour everything into a baking tin which is laid out with baking sheets.
3. Bake at 350°F for 30 minutes or until golden brown. Have an eye on it!

88. Coconut Bread

Made for: Breakfast | Prep Time: 35 minutes | Breads: 16
Per Bread: Kcal: 158, Protein: 4g, Fat: 11g, Net Carb: 6g

INGREDIENTS

- ❖ 6 organic eggs, at room temperature
- ❖ 1/2 cup (120ml) coconut oil, melted and cooled
- ❖ 3/4 cup (84g) coconut flour
- ❖ 2 tablespoons arrowroot powder
- ❖ 1/2 teaspoon sea salt
- ❖ 1 teaspoon baking powder

INSTRUCTIONS

1. Preheat oven to 350 degrees.
2. Use a medium bowl, mix eggs, coconut oil and honey.
3. Mix until all the wet ingredients are combined.
4. Add coconut flour, arrowroot powder, baking powder and salt to the wet mixture and mix until the batter is lump free.
5. Allow the batter to sit for 5 minutes.
6. Scoop batter into a greased bread pan (I used a medium bread pan, 7 3/8″ x 3 5/8″ x 2″).
7. Bake bread until the top is golden brown and a toothpick inserted into the middle comes out clean, about 35-40 minutes.

89. Carb-Free Bread

Prep Time: 35 minutes | Breads: 16
Per Breads: Kcal: 150, Protein: 5g, Fat: 9g, Net Carb: 2g

INGREDIENTS

- ❖ 2 cups (300g) flax seed

- ❖ 5 egg whites
- ❖ 2 whole eggs
- ❖ 5 tbsp. flax oil, coconut oil, or olive oil
- ❖ 1 tbsp. baking powder
- ❖ 1 teas. salt
- ❖ 1/2 cup (125ml) water
- ❖ 3 packets Stevia

INSTRUCTIONS

1. Preheat oven to 350
2. Add all ingredients to a blender or mixer.
3. Mix and add to a lightly greased bread pan.
4. Bake at 350 for 30 minutes.
5. Remove from pan. Slice and serve.

90. Bacon and Avocado

Made for: Breakfast | **Prep Time:** 25 minutes | **Servings:** 02
Per Serving: Kcal: 410, Protein: 13g, Fat: 36g, Net Carb: 7g

INGREDIENTS

- ❖ 2 eggs
- ❖ 2 tbsp heavy cream (optional)
- ❖ to taste salt
- ❖ to taste pepper
- ❖ 2 tsp butter
- ❖ 2 tbsp mayonnaise
- ❖ 1 cup (48g) romaine lettuce (chopped)
- ❖ 1 roma tomato (sliced)
- ❖ 4 cooked bacon strips
- ❖ 1/2 avocado (sliced)

INSTRUCTIONS

1. Whisk the eggs well with the heavy cream, salt and pepper.
2. Heat up a non-stick pan to a medium heat.
3. Melt half the butter in the pan, and pour in half the egg mixture. Immediately tilt the pan back and forth to ensure the egg covers the entire base.
4. Cover the pan and let the cook for about a minute.
5. When you are able to move the entire crepe when shaking the pan back and forth, carefully flip it over with a spatula.
6. When it's fully cooked, transfer to a paper towel to remove excess oiliness.

7. Repeat with the other half of the egg mix.
8. Spread the mayonaisse on the crepe.
9. Add the lettuce, tomato, bacon and avocado.
10. Season with salt and pepper.
11. Roll and enjoy!

91. Keto Scrambled Eggs

Made for: Breakfast | **Prep Time:** 10 minutes | **Servings:** 01
Per Serving: Kcal: 390, Protein: 19g, Fat: 32g, Net Carb: 3g

INGREDIENTS

- ❖ 2 large Egg
- ❖ 1 tablespoon Unsalted Butter to cook eggs
- ❖ 1/8 teaspoon salt
- ❖ 1/4 cup (20g) Grated Cheddar
- ❖ 1/4 cup (38g) Avocado
- ❖ 1/4 diced Tomato

INSTRUCTIONS

1. In a medium mixing bowl, whisk eggs with salt and pepper
2. Heat a non-stick skillet over medium-high heat with butter
3. When the butter has just melted (not brown) pour in the beaten eggs, layer cheese on top, and reduce to medium heat.
4. Let the eggs cook for 30 seconds (no stirring!) then gently move a spatula across the bottom and side of the skillet to broken up eggs and form a soft egg curd.
5. Stop stirring and cook again for 15 seconds to set.
6. Repeat this process of stirring and cooking until the eggs thickened, slightly set but still soft and runny in some places.
7. Serve immediately on a slice of keto bread loaf or on its own with diced avocado, diced tomatoes, and chives. Feel free to add other toppings like crispy bacon, sour cream, or fried mushrooms.

92. Keto Egg Wraps

Made for: Breakfast | **Prep Time:** 15 minutes | **Servings:** 04
Per Serving: Kcal: 70, Protein: 24g, Fat: 6g, Net Carb: 1g

INGREDIENTS

- ❖ Avocado Oil or other oil for greasing pan
- ❖ 4 Eggs (or 1 egg per wrap for small/ mediums pans 6-8 inches & 2 eggs for large pans 10-12 inches)
- ❖ Salt + Pepper

INSTRUCTIONS

1. Lightly grease a 6-8 inch non stick skillet with oil and warm over a medium heat.
2. While the pan in heating, whisk one egg in a small cup or bowl.
3. After the pan has fully heated up, pour in the whisked egg. Swirl the pan around or use a spoon to spread the egg evenly across the bottom of the pan to form a full circle. Sprinkle a pinch of salt and pepper across the top of the egg as it cooks.
4. Let cook 30-60 seconds until the edges are cooked then gently flip over to cook on the other side And cook another 30-60 seconds.
5. Transfer the egg to a plate to cool and then repeat with the remaining eggs.
6. Once made these wraps can be kept 1-2 days.

93. Keto Breakfast Muffins

Made for: Breakfast | **Prep Time:** 5 minutes | **Cups:** 12
Per Cups: Kcal: 197, Protein: 15g, Fat: 36g, Net Carb: 2g

INGREDIENTS

- ❖ ⅔ cup/108g cottage cheese
- ❖ ½ cup/45g grated parmesan cheese
- ❖ ¼ cup/28g coconut flour
- ❖ ⅔ cup/75g almond flour
- ❖ 1 teaspoon baking powder
- ❖ ½ teaspoon salt
- ❖ 3 tablespoons water
- ❖ 5 eggs beaten
- ❖ 3 strips no sugar bacon cooked until crisp, fat blotted with paper towel, then crumbled
- ❖ ½ cup/56g cheddar cheese shredded

INSTRUCTIONS

1. Preheat oven to 400 F. Spray or grease muffin cups.

2. In mixing bowl, combine cottage cheese, parmesan cheese, coconut flour, almond meal, baking powder, salt, water, and beaten egg. Mix in crumbled bacon and cheddar cheese.
3. Fill muffin cups ½ to ¾ full. Sprinkle muffin tops with additional shredded cheddar cheese, if desired. Bake 25 -30 minutes, until muffins are firm and lightly browned. Can be served hot or at room temperature.

94. Sheet Pan Breakfast

Made for: Breakfast | **Prep Time:** 5 minutes | **Servings:** 01
Per Serving: Kcal: 320, Protein: 0g, Fat: 36g, Net Carb: 0g

INGREDIENTS

- ❖ 1 tbsp MCT Oil
- ❖ 2 tbsp Butter
- ❖ 12 oz Coffee

INSTRUCTIONS

1. Brew a cup of coffee using any brewing method you'd like.
2. Add butter, MCT oil, and coffee to a blender. Blend on high for 30 seconds. Enjoy.

95. Bacon Egg and Cheese

Made for: Breakfast | **Prep Time:** 10 minutes | **Servings:** 01
Per Serving: Kcal: 589, Protein: 28g, Fat: 89g, Net Carb: 3g

INGREDIENTS

- ❖ 2 slices homemade keto white bread
- ❖ 1 slice cheddar cheese
- ❖ 2 slices bacon cooked until crispy
- ❖ 1 egg fried

INSTRUCTIONS

1. Place the cheese on top of the slice of bread, and broil until the cheese is melted (stay with it, this happens fast!).
2. Top with the bacon, egg, and microgreens (if using).
3. Serve.

96. Egg & Sausage Breakfast

Made for: Breakfast | **Prep Time:** 45 minutes | **Servings:** 02
Per Serving: Kcal: 375, Protein: 21 g, Fat: 32g, Net Carbs: 2 g

INGREDIENTS

- ❖ 12 eggs.
- ❖ 8 oz breakfast sausage.
- ❖ 8 oz cheddar cheese (grated).
- ❖ ¾ cup/180ml of thick cream/double cream
- ❖ 1 tbsp onion (grated).
- ❖ 2 tsp mustard (powder).
- ❖ 1 tsp oregano (dried).

INSTRUCTIONS

1. Preheat oven at 350.
2. In a large frying pan, fry sausage for 6-7 minutes, breaking it with a fork as it cooks,
3. eventually looking like a crumble mixture. Spread into a casserole dish.
4. In a bowl, mix eggs, cheese, onion, oregano, mustard, and cream until well
5. combined. Pour over sausage mixture.
6. Bake for 35-40 minutes until thoroughly cooked.

97. Bacon & Broccoli Wrap

Made for: Breakfast | **Prep Time:** 5 minutes | **Servings:** 02
Per Serving: Kcal: 258, Protein: 15g, Fat: 19g, Net Carb: 4g

INGREDIENTS

- ❖ One large egg.
- ❖ One cup broccoli (chopped).
- ❖ One onion (sliced).
- ❖ One slice of bacon.
- ❖ ¼ cup/50g tomatoes (chopped).
- ❖ 2 tbsp cheddar cheese.
- ❖ 1 tbsp milk.
- ❖ 1 tsp avocado oil.
- ❖ Pinch salt and pepper.

INSTRUCTIONS

1. Fry bacon until crispy and remove from pan. Add broccoli and cook for 3 minutes until soft, mix in tomatoes and pour into a bowl.
2. In a separate bowl, mix egg, milk, onion, and salt and pepper. Add oil to a large frying

3. pan over medium heat; pour in the egg mixture, covering the frying pan's base. Cook for 2 minutes until the bottom has set, flip and cook the other side.
4. Place egg wrap on a plate, fill the bottom half with broccoli mixture, top with bacon, and roll into a wrap.

98. Coconut Milk Shake

Made for: Breakfast | **Prep Time:** 15 minutes | **Servings:** 01
Per Serving: Kcal: 224, Protein: 16g, Fat: 44g, Net Carb: 0.2g

INGREDIENTS

- ❖ ½ avocado
- ❖ ½ cups/120ml Unsweetened Coconut Milk
- ❖ 5 drops stevia
- ❖ 5 Ice Cubes

INSTRUCTIONS

1. Add all the ingredients to the blender.
2. Blend until smooth.

99. Strawberry Pancakes

Made for: Breakfast | **Prep Time:** 15 minutes | **Servings:** 04
Per Serving: Kcal: 320, Protein: 14g, Fat: 36g, Net Carb: 4g

INGREDIENTS

- ❖ Four large eggs.
- ❖ 1 cup of thick cream.
- ❖ 7 oz cottage cheese.
- ❖ 2 oz fresh strawberries.
- ❖ 2 oz butter.
- ❖ 1 tbsp psyllium husk (powder).

INSTRUCTIONS

1. Mix cottage cheese, eggs, and psyllium husk until well combined. Allow resting for 10 minutes.
2. Heat butter in a large frying pan and fry each pancake on medium heat for 3-4 minutes on each side.
3. In a bowl, whip the cream until peaks are formed.
4. Serve the pancakes topped with cream and fresh strawberries.

100. Coconut Porridge

Made for: Breakfast | **Prep Time:** 15 minutes | **Servings:** 01
Per Serving: Kcal: 444, Protein: 10g, Fat: 36g, Net Carb: 6g

INGREDIENTS

- ❖ ½ cup (120 ml) almond milk.
- ❖ ¼ cup (35 g) of mixed berries.
- ❖ ⅓ cup (75 ml) of coconut milk.
- ❖ 2 tbsp flaxseed.
- ❖ 1 tbsp desiccated coconut.
- ❖ 1 tbsp almond meal.
- ❖ 1 tsp pumpkin seeds.
- ❖ ½ tsp cinnamon.
- ❖ ½ tsp vanilla extract.

INSTRUCTIONS

1. To a large saucepan, add coconut milk, almond milk, flaxseed, almond meal, coconut, cinnamon, and vanilla; stir continuously until mixture thickens.
2. Pour into a bowl and top with pumpkin seeds and mixed fruit.

Keto Lunch Recipes

101. Creamy Garlic Chicken

Made for: lunch | **Prep Time:** 25 minutes | **Servings:** 02
Per Serving: Kcal: 378, Protein: 10g, Fat: 26g, Net Carb: 7g

INGREDIENTS

- ❖ 1½ pounds (700g) boneless skinless chicken breasts thinly sliced
- ❖ 2 Tablespoons olive oil
- ❖ 1 cup heavy cream/double cream
- ❖ 1/2 cup/50g chicken broth
- ❖ One teaspoon garlic powder
- ❖ One teaspoon Italian seasoning
- ❖ 1/2 cup/45g parmesan cheese
- ❖ 1 cup/30g spinach chopped
- ❖ 1/2 cup/26g sun-dried tomatoes

INSTRUCTIONS

1. In a large skillet, add olive oil and cook the chicken on medium-high heat for 3-5 minutes on each side or until brown on each side and cooked until no longer pink in centre. Remove chicken and set aside on a plate.
2. Add the heavy cream, chicken broth, garlic powder, Italian seasoning, and parmesan cheese. Whisk over medium-high heat until it starts to thicken. Add the spinach and sundried tomatoes and let it simmer until the spinach begins to wilt. Add the chicken back to the pan and serve over pasta if desired.

102. Garlic Butter Steak

Made for: lunch | **Prep Time:** 15 minutes | **Servings:** 04
Per Serving: Kcal: 461, Protein: 5g, Fat: 31g, Net Carb: 2g

INGREDIENTS:

- ❖ Six medium cloves garlic
- ❖ kosher salt
- ❖ 1.5 lb. skirt steak, trimmed and cut into four pieces
- ❖ freshly ground Black Pepper
- ❖ Two tablespoons canola oil or vegetable oil
- ❖ 2 oz. unsalted butter (4 tablespoons)
- ❖ One tablespoon chopped fresh flat-leaf parsley

INSTRUCTIONS

1. Peel the garlic cloves and smash them with the side of a chef's knife. Sprinkle the garlic lightly with salt and mince it.
2. Pat the steak dry and season generously on both sides with salt and Pepper. In a heavy-duty 12-inch skillet, heat the oil over medium-high heat until shimmering hot. Add the steak and brown well on both sides, 2 to 3 minutes per side for medium-rare. Transfer the steak to a plate and let rest while you make the garlic butter.
3. In an 8-inch skillet, melt the butter over low heat. Add the garlic and cook, swirling the pan frequently, until lightly golden, about 4 minutes. Lightly salt to taste.
4. Slice the steak, if you like, and transfer to 4 plates. Spoon the garlic butter over the steak, sprinkle with the parsley, and serve.

103. Keto Guacamole

Made for: lunch | **Prep Time:** 10 minutes | **Servings:** 01
Per Serving: Kcal: 238, Protein: 3g, Fat: 21g, Net Carb: 5g

INGREDIENTS

- ❖ 1 avocado ripe
- ❖ ½ lime juiced
- ❖ 1 clove garlic minced or grated
- ❖ ⅛ tsp cumin ground
- ❖ salt to taste

INSTRUCTIONS

1. Cut avocado in half and discard pit. Scoop out avocado flesh and place in a bowl or mortar.
2. Add lime juice, garlic, cumin, and salt. If you want smooth guacamole, add any optional mix-ins.
3. Using a pestle or fork, crush ingredients together until you reach desired consistency.
4. If you prefer a chunky-style guacamole, add optional mix-ins once avocado has been mashed.

104. Spicy Shrimp

Made for: lunch | **Prep Time:** 25 minutes | **Servings:** 02
Per Serving: Kcal: 122, Protein: 00g, Fat: 5g, Net Carb: 3g

INGREDIENTS

- ❖ 1 pound peeled and deveined shrimp
- ❖ 1 tablespoon paprika
- ❖ 2 teaspoons garlic powder
- ❖ ½ teaspoon cayenne pepper
- ❖ 1 tablespoon extra-virgin olive oil
- ❖ Salt and freshly ground Black Pepper

INSTRUCTIONS

1. Place the shrimp in a large zip-top plastic bag. In a small bowl, stir the paprika with the garlic powder and cayenne to combine. Pour the mixture into the container with the shrimp and toss well until they are coated with the spices. Refrigerate while you make the grits.

105. Tomatoes and Cheese

Made for: lunch | **Prep Time:** 25 minutes | **Servings:** 02
Per Serving: Kcal: 435, Protein: 26.5g, Fat: 32g, Net Carb: 1g

INGREDIENTS

- ❖ Six large eggs
- ❖ 1/2 medium or yellow-white onion (55 g)
- ❖ 2/3 cup crumbled soft cheese like feta
- ❖ 2/3 cup (100 g) cherry tomatoes, halved
- ❖ 1 tbsp ghee or duck fat (15 ml)
- ❖ 2 tbsp freshly chopped herbs such as chives or basil
- ❖ sea salt and ground pepper, to taste

INSTRUCTIONS

1. Preheat the oven (or ideally grill if you have it) to 200 °C / 400 °F (fan assisted), or 220 °C / 425 °F (conventional). Peel and slice the onion. Place on a hot pan greased with ghee and cook until lightly browned.
2. Crack the eggs into a bowl and season with salt and Pepper. Add finely chopped herbs (I used chives) and whisk well.
3. When the onion is browned, pour in the eggs and cook until you see the edges turning opaque.
4. Top with the crumbled cheese and halved cherry tomatoes. Place under the broiler and cook for 5-7 minutes or until the top is cooked.
5. Remove from the oven and set aside to cool down. Serve immediately or store in the fridge for up to 5 days. You can freeze the frittata fr up to 3 months.

106. Keto Egg Loaf

Made for: lunch | **Prep Time:** 15 minutes | **Servings:** 12 Slice
Per Slice: Kcal: 177, Protein: 6g, Fat: 14g, Net Carb: 5g

INGREDIENTS

- ❖ 8 large Eggs
- ❖ 8 oz Cream Cheese full-fat
- ❖ ½ cup (55g) Coconut Flour
- ❖ 4 tablespoon Butter unsalted, melted

❖ 1 teaspoon Baking Powder

INSTRUCTIONS

1. Preheat the oven to 350°F and line a 9x5-inch loaf pan with parchment paper.
2. In a large mixing bowl combine the eggs with the melted butter and cream cheese. Whisk until they turn into a smooth batter.
3. Fold in the baking powder and coconut flour.
4. Pour the batter in the prepared loaf pan and bake in the preheated oven for 45-50 minutes, until golden brown.
5. Let it reach room temperature before removing from the loaf pan, slice and serve.

107. Chewy Coconut Chunks

Made for: lunch | **Prep Time:** 25 minutes | **Servings:** 08
Per Serving: Kcal: 111, Protein: 2g, Fat: 10g, Net Carb: 7g

INGREDIENTS

❖ 7 oz coconut (shredded).
❖ ⅔ cup/160ml coconut milk (full fat).
❖ ¼ cup/40g Erythritol
❖ 1 tsp psyllium husk.
❖ ¼ tsp almond extract.
❖ ¼ tsp salt.

INSTRUCTIONS

1. Preheat oven at 325 degrees.
2. In a blender, mix coconut milk, maple syrup, psyllium husk, almond extract, salt, and ¾ of the coconut flakes until smooth.
3. Pour mixture into a large bowl, stir in remaining coconut flakes.
4. Line a baking tray with greaseproof paper. Using a tablespoon, scoop out chunks of the mixture and place onto the plate.
5. Bake for 30 minutes or until all chunks are golden brown.

108. Keto Carrot Cake

Made for: lunch | **Prep Time:** 20 minutes | **Servings:** 02
Per Serving: Kcal: 443, Protein: 14g, Fat: 40g, Net Carb: 5g

INGREDIENTS

❖ ¾ cup/85g almond flour.
❖ ½ cup/25g carrot (grated).
❖ One large egg.
❖ 2 tbsp cream cheese.
❖ 2 tbsp walnuts (finely chopped).
❖ 2 tbsp butter (melted).
❖ 2 tbsp erythritol.
❖ 1 tbsp thick cream or double cream.
❖ 2 tsp cinnamon.
❖ 1 tsp mixed spice.
❖ 1 tsp baking powder.

INSTRUCTIONS

1. In a bowl, mix almond flour, cinnamon, baking powder, erythritol, walnuts, and mixed spice.
2. Mix in the egg, butter, thick cream, and carrot until well combined.
3. Grease 2 microwave-safe ramekins and split the mixture evenly between the two.
4. Microwave on high for 5 minutes.
5. Spread cream cheese on the top.

109. Mozzarella Chicken

Made for: lunch | **Prep Time:** 25 minutes | **Servings:** 04
Per Serving: Kcal: 342, Protein: 31g, Fat: 24g, Net Carb: 0.9g

INGREDIENTS

❖ Four small chicken breasts
❖ One tablespoon olive oil
❖ One tablespoon minced garlic
❖ ½ cup/80g chopped onions
❖ 1 (14 ounces) can crushed tomatoes
❖ ½ teaspoon EACH Italian seasoning AND red pepper flakes (see notes)
❖ ¼ teaspoon dried basil
❖ One tablespoon sun-dried tomato pesto (homemade
❖ salt and pepper + ¼ cup water
❖ Four slices mozzarella cheese (or 1 cup shredded)

INSTRUCTIONS

1. CHICKEN: Sprinkle the chicken with a pinch

of salt and pepper on both sides. Heat a large nonstick skillet over medium-high heat with the olive oil. Add the chicken to the skillet and cook for about 3-5 minutes per side or until the chicken is thoroughly cooked through, remove to a plate. If you are planning on serving this with pasta, get the water going and cook the pasta according to package directions.

2. TOMATO SAUCE: Preheat the oven on the broiler setting. Add the onions to the oil remaining in the pan. If there isn't any, add in about ½ teaspoon and sauté the onion for 2-3 minutes until they soften, add the garlic and let cook for 30 seconds. Add the crushed tomatoes, Italian seasoning, red pepper flakes, dried basil, and pesto and stir to combine. When the sauce reaches a simmer, add a ¼ cup of water, lower the heat, cover and allow to simmer for 10-12 minutes or until the sauce thickens a bit— season with salt and Pepper to taste.

3. ASSEMBLE: Nestle the chicken breasts into the sauce and using a spoon, cover the chicken with seasoning. Top each breast with a slice of cheese. Place under the broiler for 1-2 minutes or until the cheese gets friendly and bubbly and just melts. Top with chopped parsley or basil ribbons. Serve with pasta or crusty bread and a salad.

110. Almond & Vanilla Keto

Made for: lunch | **Prep Time:** 15 minutes | **Servings:** 02
Per Serving: Kcal: 435, Protein: 9g, Fat: 43g, Net Carb: 6g

INGREDIENTS

- ❖ 16 oz cream cheese.
- ❖ 2 cups almond flour.
- ❖ One ¼ cup (25 g) erythritol.
- ❖ ¾ cup (180 ml) of thick cream/double cream
- ❖ ½ cup (120 g) sour cream.
- ❖ ⅓ cup (80 g) butter (melted).
- ❖ 2 tsp vanilla extract.

INSTRUCTIONS

1. Mix butter, flour, ¼ cup erythritol, and 1 tsp vanilla until a dough is formed.
2. Press the dough into a 9-inch ovenproof dish and chill for 60 minutes.
3. In a blender, mix cream cheese, 1 cup erythritol, and remaining vanilla until creamy.
4. Add in the sour cream and thick cream until thickened.
5. Pour onto chilled crust and refrigerate for 4-5 hours.

111. Garlic Shrimp Zoodles

Made for: lunch | **Prep Time:** 20 minutes | **Servings:** 04
Per Serving: Kcal: 353, Protein: 14g, Fat: 10g, Net Carb: 9g

INGREDIENTS

- ❖ Two medium zucchini/Courgette
- ❖ 3/4 pounds medium shrimp peeled & deveined
- ❖ One tablespoon olive oil
- ❖ Juice and zest of 1 lemon
- ❖ 3-4 cloves garlic minced
- ❖ Red pepper flakes (optional)
- ❖ Salt & Pepper to taste
- ❖ Chopped fresh parsley

INSTRUCTIONS

1. Spiralize the zucchini on the medium setting. Set aside.
2. Add the olive oil and lemon juice & zest to a skillet on medium heat. Once the pan is warm, add the shrimp—Cook, the shrimp for one minute per side.
3. Add the garlic and red pepper flakes. Cook for an additional minute, stirring often.
4. Add the zucchini noodles and stir/toss (e.g., with tongs) regularly for 2-3 minutes until they're slightly cooked and warmed up.
5. Season with salt and pepper and sprinkle with the chopped parsley. Serve immediately

112. Garlic Gnocchi

Made for: lunch | **Prep Time:** 15 minutes | **Servings:** 04
Per Serving: Kcal: 314, Protein: 13g, Fat: 27g, Net Carb: 7g

INGREDIENTS

- ❖ 1 ⅓ cup (150g) almond flour.
- ❖ ⅔ cup (60g) parmesan (grated).
- ❖ ½ cup (130g) ricotta cheese.
- ❖ One large egg.
- ❖ Four garlic cloves (chopped).
- ❖ 2 tbsp coconut flour.
- ❖ 2 tbsp butter.
- ❖ 2 tbsp olive oil.
- ❖ 2 tsp xanthan gum.
- ❖ 1 tsp garlic powder.
- ❖ ¼ tsp salt.

INSTRUCTIONS

1. In a bowl, mix almond flour, coconut flour, garlic powder, and xanthan gum.
2. In a separate bowl, whisk the egg and add ricotta, parmesan, and salt; mix until well combined.
3. Add the flour mixture to the cheese mixture and mix thoroughly until the crumble becomes a sticky dough ball.
4. Wrap the dough ball in cling film and let settle in the fridge for 60 minutes.
5. Cut the dough into 1-inch pieces, moulding them into an oval shape.
6. In a large frying pan, add olive oil and butter; fry the garlic until lightly browned.
7. Fry the gnocchi for 5 minutes, spooning on the garlic oil.

113. Tangy & Tasty BBQ Pork

Made for: lunch | **Prep Time:** 20 minutes | **Servings:** 02
Per Serving: Kcal: 999, Protein: 53g, Fat: 80g, Net Carb: 6g

INGREDIENTS

- ❖ 48 oz pork ribs.
- ❖ ¼ cup (60g) dijon mustard.
- ❖ 4 tbsp paprika powder.
- ❖ 2 tbsp butter.
- ❖ 2 tbsp apple cider vinegar.
- ❖ 2 tbsp garlic powder.
- ❖ 1 ½ tbsp black pepper.
- ❖ 1 tbsp salt.
- ❖ 1 tbsp chilli powder.
- ❖ 2 tsp onion powder.

INSTRUCTIONS

1. Preheat oven at 400 degrees.
2. In a bowl, mix mustard and vinegar.
3. In a separate bowl, mix paprika, garlic, pepper, salt, chilli, and onion powder.
4. Have a large sheet of foil next to both bowls. Dip each rib into the vinegar mixture (ensure both sides are covered) then dip into the spice mixture (provide bones are completely covered)—place ribs on the foil.
5. Add the butter to the top of the ribs. Wrap the ribs in foil (use another piece to secure).
6. Place ribs on a baking tray and bake for 60 minutes.
7. When ribs are ready, remove from oven and foil.
8. Grill on high heat to give additional colour.

114. Zucchini Pizza Boats

Made for: lunch | **Prep Time:** 25 minutes | **Servings:** 02
Per Serving: Kcal: 345, Protein: 31g, Fat: 17g, Net Carb: 7g

INGREDIENTS

- ❖ Four zucchinis/ Courgettes, sliced in half lengthwise
- ❖ One small can Pizza Sauce
- ❖ 1/2 8oz package button mushrooms, sliced
- ❖ One small red onion, diced
- ❖ 1/2 green pepper, diced
- ❖ 2 cups shredded mozzarella cheese
- ❖ 1 tbsp fresh chopped basil (optional topping)
- ❖ 1 tsp red chilli flakes (optional topping)
- ❖ 2 tsp olive oil
- ❖ 1/2 lb ground turkey
- ❖ 2 tsp fennel seeds
- ❖ 1 tsp garlic powder
- ❖ 1/2 tsp salt
- ❖ 1 tsp Italian seasoning

INSTRUCTIONS

1. Preheat olive oil in a large skillet over med-high heat. Add turkey and seasonings, crushing up with a crushing spoon and mixing well. Cook for 5-6 minutes until

turkey is browned and fully cooked. Remove from heat and set aside.

2. Preheat oven to 400 F. Cut zucchini in half lengthwise and scoop out the flesh. On a baking sheet or in a 9x13 casserole dish, spread each zucchini boat with pizza sauce, then top with sausage, mushrooms, red onion, green pepper, and cheese.
3. Bake in the oven for 15 minutes or until cheese is melted. Remove from oven and sprinkle with fresh basil and chilli flakes. Serve and enjoy!

115. Keto chicken enchilada

Made for: lunch | **Prep Time:** 25 minutes | **Servings:** 04
Per Serving: Kcal: 568, Protein: 38g, Fat: 40g, Net Carb: 6g

INGREDIENTS

- ❖ Two tablespoon coconut oil (for searing chicken)
- ❖ 1 pound of boneless, skinless chicken thighs
- ❖ 3/4 cup (195g) red enchilada sauce (recipe from Low Carb Maven)
- ❖ 1/4 cup (65ml) water
- ❖ 1/4 cup (28g) chopped onion
- ❖ 1– 4 oz can dice green chiles

INSTRUCTIONS

1. In a pot or dutch oven over medium heat, melt the coconut oil. Once hot, sear chicken thighs until lightly brown.
2. Pour in enchilada sauce and water, then add onion and green chiles. Reduce heat to a simmer and cover. Cook chicken for 17-25 minutes or until chicken is tender and fully cooked through to at least 165 degrees internal temperature.
3. Carefully removes the chicken and place it onto a work surface. Chop or shred chicken (your preference), then add it back into the pot. Let the chicken simmer uncovered for an additional 10 minutes to absorb flavour and allow the sauce to reduce a little.
4. To serve, top with avocado, cheese, jalapeno, sour cream, tomato, and any other desired toppings. Feel free to customize these to your preference. Serve alone or over

cauliflower rice, if desired, just be sure to update your nutrition info as needed.

116. Sassy Pork Stir-fry

Made for: lunch | **Prep Time:** 25 minutes | **Servings:** 04
Per Serving: Kcal: 225, Protein: 17g, Fat: 14g, Net Carb: 9g

INGREDIENTS

- ❖ 12 oz pork loin (chopped into strips).
- ❖ 12 oz broccoli (florets).
- ❖ Six spring onions (chopped).
- ❖ One red pepper (sliced).
- ❖ 2 tbsp olive oil.
- ❖ 2 tbsp soy sauce.
- ❖ 1 ½ tbsp coconut sugar.
- ❖ 1 tbsp garlic (crushed).
- ❖ 1 tbsp dry sherry.
- ❖ 1 tsp sesame oil.

INSTRUCTIONS

1. Mix 1 tbsp olive oil with the crushed garlic; dip each strip of pork in the mixture.
2. In a large frying pan, add the remaining olive oil and fry the pork until cooked through.
3. Remove pork from pan. In the same frying pan, load in the broccoli, onions, and red pepper; stir and cover for 1 minute.
4. In a bowl, mix sherry, sesame oil, soy sauce, and coconut sugar.
5. Add pork and any juices to the vegetables and stir well.
6. Pour sherry mixture over the pork and vegetables.
7. Fry until sauce thickens.

117. Shrimp & Sausage

Made for: lunch | **Prep Time:** 25 minutes | **Servings:** 04
Per Serving: Kcal: 750, Protein: 17g, Fat: 32g, Net Carb: 4g

INGREDIENTS

- ❖ 1 lb of medium or large shrimp (peeled and deveined)
- ❖ 6 oz of pre-cooked smoked sausage, chopped (choose your favourite)
- ❖ 3/4 cup/110g diced red bell pepper

- ❖ 3/4 cup (110g) diced green bell pepper
- ❖ 1/2 of a medium yellow onion, diced
- ❖ 1/4 cup/120ml chicken stock
- ❖ One zucchini/Courgette, chopped
- ❖ Two garlic cloves, diced
- ❖ Salt & Pepper to taste
- ❖ Pinch of red pepper flakes
- ❖ 2 tsp Old Bay Seasoning
- ❖ Olive oil or coconut oil
- ❖ Optional garnish: chopped parsley

INSTRUCTIONS

1. Heat a large skillet over medium-high heat with some olive oil or coconut oil
2. Season shrimp with Old Bay Seasoning
3. Cook shrimp about 3-4 minutes until opaque – remove and set aside
4. Cook onions and bell peppers in skillet with 2 Tbsp of olive oil or coconut oil for about 2 minutes
5. Add sausage and zucchini to the skillet, cook another 2 minutes
6. Put cooked shrimp back into the skillet along with the garlic, and cook everything for about 1 minute
7. Pour chicken stock into the pan and mix through to moisten everything
8. Add salt, ground pepper, and red pepper flakes to taste
9. Remove from heat, garnish with parsley and serve hot

118. Keto Chili Kicker

Made for: lunch | **Prep Time:** 20 minutes | **Servings:** 02
Per Serving: Kcal: 330, Protein: 35g, Fat: 15g, Net Carb: 4g

INGREDIENTS

- ❖ 16 oz minced beef.
- ❖ Two avocados (chopped).
- ❖ One tomato (finely chopped).
- ❖ One garlic clove (crushed).
- ❖ 3 tbsp lime juice (fresh).
- ❖ 2 tbsp red onion (finely chopped).
- ❖ 1 tbsp coriander (ground).
- ❖ 1 tbsp cumin (ground).
- ❖ ½ tsp cayenne pepper.
- ❖ ½ tsp garlic powder.

- ❖ ¼ tsp black pepper.

INSTRUCTIONS

1. In a large frying pan, add minced beef, coriander, cumin, cayenne pepper, and garlic powder. Fry for 6-8 minutes or until meat is thoroughly cooked.
2. In a bowl, mix avocados, tomatoes, crushed garlic, onion, lime juice, and black pepper; mix until well combined.
3. Put chilli into a bowl and serve avocado salsa on top.

119. Salmon Lemon Sauce

Made for: lunch | **Prep Time:** 20 minutes | **Servings:** 04
Per Serving: Kcal: 352, Protein: 28g, Fat: 22g, Net Carb: 9g

INGREDIENTS

- ❖ 4 (5 ounces) salmon fillets, skins removed
- ❖ salt and Pepper to taste
- ❖ 1 (12 ounces) container ricotta
- ❖ 1/2 cup (45 g) Parmigiano Reggiano (parmesan), grated
- ❖ Two tablespoons basil, chopped
- ❖ Two teaspoons lemon zest
- ❖ salt and Pepper to taste
- ❖ 1/2 pound asparagus, trimmed
- ❖ One tablespoon butter
- ❖ 1/2 cup (50 g) chicken broth
- ❖ Two tablespoons lemon juice
- ❖ Two teaspoons cornstarch

INSTRUCTIONS

1. Season the salmon fillets with salt and Pepper to taste, lay them down with the skin side up, top with the mixture of the ricotta, parmesan, basil, lemon zest, salt and Pepper, several spears of asparagus and roll them up before placing them on a greased baking sheet with the seam side down.
2. Bake in a preheated 425F/220C oven until the salmon is just cooked, about 15-20 minutes.
3. Meanwhile, melt the butter in a small saucepan over medium heat, add the mixture of the broth, lemon juice, and corn

starch and heat until it thickens, about 3-5 minutes.

4. Serve the salmon rolls topped with the lemon sauce and optionally garnish with more basil and lemon zest.

120. Coconut Chicken Curry

Made for: lunch | **Prep Time:** 25 minutes | **Servings:** 04
Per Serving: Kcal: 465, Protein: 28g, Fat: 30g, Net Carb: 6g

INGREDIENTS

- ❖ 27 oz coconut milk.
- ❖ 16 oz chicken thighs (boneless and skinless, cubed).
- ❖ 8 oz broccoli (cut into small florets).
- ❖ 3 oz green beans (cut in half).
- ❖ One onion (finely chopped).
- ❖ One chilli pepper (finely chopped).
- ❖ 3 tbsp coconut oil.
- ❖ 1 tbsp fresh ginger (grated).
- ❖ 1 tbsp curry paste.
- ❖ Salt and Pepper.

Cauliflower rice:

- ❖ 24 oz cauliflower head (grated).
- ❖ 3 oz coconut oil.
- ❖ ½ tsp salt.

INSTRUCTIONS

1. Heat coconut oil in a frying pan. Add onion, chilli, and ginger and fry until softened.
2. Add chicken and curry paste; fry until chicken is cooked and lightly browned.
3. Add broccoli and green beans.
4. Add the substantial part of coconut milk, salt, and Pepper. Allow simmering for 15-20 minutes.
5. In another large frying pan, add 3 oz coconut oil. When hot, add the grated cauliflower.
6. Add salt and cook for 5-10 minutes until rice has softened.
7. Place rice on a serving plate and top with chicken curry.

121. Luscious Cheesy Choice

Made for: lunch | **Prep Time:** 15 minutes | **Servings:** 04
Per Serving: Kcal: 633, Protein: 48g, Fat: 44g, Net Carb: 9g

INGREDIENTS

Cheese dough:
- ❖ 1 ½ cups mozzarella (grated).
- ❖ 4 oz cream cheese (softened).
- ❖ Two large eggs.
- ❖ 1 tsp mixed herbs (dried).

Filling:
- ❖ 16 oz minced beef.
- ❖ One red onion (finely chopped).
- ❖ One cup mozzarella (grated).
- ❖ 1 cup marinara sauce.
- ❖ 6 tbsp ricotta cheese.
- ❖ 1 tsp mixed herbs (dried)
- ❖ Salt and Pepper.

INSTRUCTIONS

1. Preheat oven at 350 degrees.
2. Add all dough ingredients to a blender; blend until a thick, smooth consistency is formed.
3. Line a 9 x 12-inch ovenproof dish with greaseproof paper.
4. Use a spatula to spread the dough mixture evenly across the dish.
5. Bake for 20-25 minutes or until the mixture is firm to the touch. Set aside and allow to cool.
6. In a large frying pan, add the beef, Salt, Pepper, and onion. Cook until completely browned.
7. Stir in marinara sauce and dried herbs; reduce heat and simmer for 5 minutes.
8. In an 8 x 4 inch ovenproof dish, add a layer of the meat mixture and place one slice of dough on top.
9. On top of the dough, add another layer of meat mixture and spread 3 tbsp of ricotta cheese on top; sprinkle ¼ cup mozzarella over.
10. Repeat with the second dough sheet, meat mixture, ricotta, and mozzarella.

11. Add last dough sheet, add remaining meat mixture, and top with remaining mozzarella.
12. Bake for 25 minutes or until the top begins to brown.

122. Chicken Lettuce Wraps

Made for: lunch | **Prep Time:** 20 minutes | **Servings:** 04
Per Serving: Kcal: 541, Protein: 44g, Fat: 28g, Net Carb: 7g

INGREDIENTS

* 1 lb ground chicken
* 1 tbsp olive oil
* 2 tbsp red curry paste
* 1 tbsp ginger minced
* Four cloves garlic minced
* One red bell pepper sliced thinly
* Four green onions chopped
* 1 cup cabbage shredded or coleslaw mix
* 1/4 cup/64g hoisin sauce
* 1/4 tsp salt or to taste
* 1/4 tsp pepper or to taste
* Five leaves basil chopped
* 1/2 head iceberg lettuce cut into half

INSTRUCTIONS

1. Add olive oil to a large skillet and heat until oil is boiling. Add ground chicken and cook until no longer pink and starts to brown, break it up with a wooden spoon as necessary. It should take about 3 minutes.
2. Add red curry paste, ginger, garlic, peppers, coleslaw mix, and stir-fry for another 3 minutes. Add hoisin sauce and green onions, and toss. Remove from heat then add basil and toss. Transfer cooked chicken to a bowl.
3. Serve by placing spoonful's of chicken into pieces of lettuce, fold lettuce over like small tacos, and eat.

123. Healthy Lunchtime Ham

Made for: lunch | **Prep Time:** 20 minutes | **Servings:** 02
Per Serving: Kcal: 459, Protein: 33g, Fat: 31g, Net Carb: 7g

INGREDIENTS

* 5 iceberg lettuce leaves.
* Four slices sandwich ham.
* 4 slices cheddar cheese.
* ¼ cup (56 g) guacamole.
* One tomato (sliced).
* ½ red onion (finely sliced.

INSTRUCTIONS

1. Layer lettuce leaves onto a sheet of cling film. Ensure the leaves overlap with each other.
2. Layer the ham and cheese onto the leaves.
3. Do the same with tomato and onion and finally top with guacamole.
4. Using the clingfilm (as if you were using a sushi mat), roll the lettuce tightly to make the wrap.
5. When completely rolled, cut the wrap in half.

124. Pancetta & Onion

Made for: lunch | **Prep Time:** 20 minutes | **Servings:** 04
Per Serving: Kcal: 885, Protein: 26g, Fat: 82g, Net Carb: 3g

INGREDIENTS

Crust:
* 1 ½ cups (170g) almond flour.
* 2 oz butter.
* One large egg.
* 2 tbsp sesame seed.
* 1 tbsp psyllium husk powder.
* ½ tsp salt.

Filling:
* Five large eggs.
* 11 oz pancetta (chopped).
* 8 oz cheddar cheese (grated).
* One onion.
* One cup of thick cream.
* 1 oz butter.
* 1 tsp thyme (dried).
* ½ tsp salt.
* ½ tsp black pepper.

INSTRUCTIONS

1. Preheat oven at 350 degrees.

2. Take all of the crust ingredients and put them in a blender. Mix until a dough is formed.
3. Using a spatula, spread the dough into a springform cake tin. Allow settling in the fridge.
4. Melt the butter in a large frying pan, add the onion and pancetta and fry until both turn golden brown. Stir in thyme, salt, and Pepper.
5. Pour into set crust.
6. In a bowl, mix the remaining ingredients and pour into crust.
7. Bake for 45-50 minutes or until the egg mixture is stable and has turned golden brown.

125. Hot & Spicy Chicken

Made for: lunch | **Prep Time:** 25 minutes | **Servings:** 02
Per Serving: Kcal: 653, Protein: 50g, Fat: 26g, Net Carb: 8g

INGREDIENTS

- ❖ 15 chicken wings.
- ❖ ½ cup (120 g) chilli paste.
- ❖ ¼ cup (25 g) erythritol.
- ❖ ⅓ cup (95 g) greek yogurt (full fat).
- ❖ ¼ cup (60 g) mayonnaise.
- ❖ 2 itbsp soy isauce.
- ❖ 2 tbsp rice wine vinegar.
- ❖ 1 ½ tbsp lime juice (fresh).
- ❖ Pinch of salt.

INSTRUCTIONS

1. Mix chilli paste, erythritol, soy sauce, and vinegar.
2. Add chicken wings to the sauce mixture and ensure each side is completely coated with the sauce.
3. Chill for 2-3 hours.
4. Preheat oven at 400 degrees.
5. Bake wings for 15 minutes, turn over and bake for an additional 15 minutes.
6. On a high heated grill, brown the chicken wings for 5-6 minutes.

7. Mix greek yoghurt, mayonnaise, lime juice, and salt. Use as a dipping sauce for the chicken wings.

126. Cheesy Chicken Chunks

Made for: lunch | **Prep Time:** 15 minutes | **Servings:** 02
Per Serving: Kcal: 686, Protein: 72g, Fat: 40g, Net Carb: 5g

INGREDIENTS

- ❖ 2 large chicken breasts (cut into strips).
- ❖ One large egg.
- ❖ ¾ cup (68 g) parmesan cheese (grated).
- ❖ ¾ cup (85 g) almond flour.

INSTRUCTIONS

1. Preheat oven at 400 degrees.
2. Mix the parmesan and flour.
3. In a separate bowl, whisk the egg.
4. Dip each strip of chicken into the egg imixture iand ithen into the flour mixture. Place on a wire rack.
5. Spray chicken with cooking spray and bake for 18-20 minutes or until browned and thoroughly cooked.

127. Chunky Salsa Tacos

Made for: lunch | **Prep Time:** 20 minutes | **Servings:** 02
Per Serving: Kcal: 306, Protein: 15g, Fat: 22g, Net Carb: 3g

INGREDIENTS

- ❖ Two large avocados (cut into small chunks).
- ❖ One tomato (cut into chunks).
- ❖ ½ red onion (roughly chopped).
- ❖ ¼ cup/5g fresh coriander (finely chopped).
- ❖ One garlic clove (finely chopped).
- ❖ 3 tbsp lime juice (fresh).
- ❖ 1 tbsp jalapeno (finely chopped).
- ❖ ½ tsp salt.
- ❖ ½ tsp black pepper.

INSTRUCTIONS

1. Preheat oven at 400 degrees.
2. Line a baking tray with greaseproof paper.

3. Make six piles of cheese with a large gap between them.
4. Bake for 10 minutes until cheese is melted and golden brown. Allow to slightly cool.
5. Place a large wire rack over the sink. Carefully place each melted cheese piece on the shelf and allow the edges to hang down between the wire rack bars.
6. Let cool completely.
7. Add all of the ingredients from the filling list to a bowl and mix well until combined.
8. Take each cheesy taco shell and add the filling.

128. Creamy Avocado

Made for: lunch | **Prep Time:** 15 minutes | **Servings:** 02
Per Serving: Kcal: 207, Protein: 5g, Fat: 15g, Net Carb: 3g

INGREDIENTS

- ❖ One avocado split and pitted
- ❖ ½ cup/140g low-fat Greek yoghurt
- ❖ One clove garlic minced
- ❖ juice of 1 lime
- ❖ 2 tbsp cilantro chopped
- ❖ salt and Pepper to taste

INSTRUCTIONS

1. In a small bowl, whisk together lime juice, olive oil, garlic, chilli powder, cumin, paprika, salt, pepper, red pepper flakes. Pour into a resealable bag and add shrimp. Toss to coat and marinate for 30 minutes.
2. Preheat the grill to medium heat. Put the shrimp on skewers and place on the rack— grill on each side for about two minutes or until no longer pink.
3. To make the creamy avocado cilantro sauce add the avocado, greek yoghurt, garlic, lime, and cilantro. Pulse in a food processor until smooth. Add salt and Pepper to taste. Serve immediately with shrimp.

129. Meatballs & Squash

Made for: lunch | **Prep Time:** 15 minutes | **Servings:** 04
Per Serving: Kcal: 382, Protein: 25g, Fat: 26g, Net Carb: 8g

INGREDIENTS

- ❖ 1 medium squash.
- ❖ 16 oz minced beef.
- ❖ 1 tsp garlic powder.
- ❖ 1 tsp paprika.
- ❖ 1 tsp onion powder.
- ❖ ½ tsp black pepper.
- ❖ ½ tsp salt.
- ❖ 2 cups marinara sauce.
- ❖ ¼ cup (25g) parmesan (grated).
- ❖ ¼ cup (62g) parsley (finely chopped).

INSTRUCTIONS

1. Preheat oven at 400 degrees.
2. Pierce the squash several times with a sharp knife and microwave for 5 minutes. Turn the squash onto the other side and microwave for an additional 5 minutes.
3. Allow squash to sit for 3-4 minutes; using a sharp knife, slice the squash in half, lengthways.
4. Scoop out the seeds. Drag a fork back and forth across the flesh and place spaghetti strands into a bowl.
5. In a large bowl, mix the minced beef, garlic powder, paprika, onion powder, Black Pepper, and salt. Combine well and form 24 small meatballs.
6. Line a baking sheet with greaseproof paper and bake meatballs for 10-15 minutes or until juices run clear.
7. In a large pan, gently heat the marinara sauce. Take the cooked meatballs and place them in the simmering sauce. Simmer for 6-8 minutes.
8. Place the spaghetti on a serving plate and pour over the sauce and meatballs.
9. Garnish with chopped parsley and parmesan.

130. Spain Cheesy-Meat

Made for: lunch | **Prep Time:** 15 minutes | **Servings:** 02
Per Serving: Kcal: 944, Protein: 57g, Fat: 74g, Net Carb: 8g

INGREDIENTS

- 8 oz prosciutto (sliced).
- 8 oz chorizo (sliced).
- 4 oz cheddar cheese (cubed).
- 4 oz mozzarella (cubed).
- 4 oz cucumber (cubed).
- 2 oz red pepper (sliced).

INSTRUCTIONS

1. Arrange all items on a plate.
2. Enjoy.

131. Cloud Nine BLT

Made for: lunch | **Prep Time**: 45 minutes | **Servings**: 02
Per Serving: Kcal: 499, Protein: 12g, Fat: 48g, Net Carb: 4g

INGREDIENTS:

Bread:

- 4 ½ oz cream cheese (softened).
- Three large eggs.
- ½ tbsp psyllium husk powder.
- ½ tsp baking powder.
- Pinch of salt.

Fillings:

- 5 oz cooked bacon (grilled).
- 2 oz lettuce.
- One tomato (sliced).
- ½ cup/120g mayonnaise.

INSTRUCTIONS

1. Preheat oven at 300 degrees.
2. Crack the eggs, putting egg whites in one bowl and yolks in another.
3. Add the salt to the egg whites and whisk until stiff peaks are formed.
4. Add the cream cheese to the egg yolks and stir well. Add psyllium husk and baking powder; mix until well combined.
5. Fold the egg white mixture into the egg yolk mixture.
6. Line a baking tray with greaseproof paper.
7. Make eight dough balls and place on the tray; flatten each one.

8. Bake for 25 minutes or until golden brown.
9. Place a slice of bread (topside down) on a serving plate and spread with mayonnaise.
10. Layer the bacon, lettuce, and tomato on to the bread; add a spoon of mayonnaise and top with the final slice of bread.

132. Pepperoni Pizza

Made for: lunch | **Prep Time**: 25 minutes | **Servings**: 02
Per Serving: Kcal: 1043, Protein: 52g, Fat: 90g, Net Carb: 5g

INGREDIENTS

- 4 large eggs.
- 6 oz mozzarella (grated)

Topping:

- 3 tbsp tomato puree.
- 5 oz mozzarella (grated).
- 1 ½ oz pepperoni (sliced).
- ½ tsp dried mixed herbs.

INSTRUCTIONS

1. Preheat oven at 400 degrees.
2. Mix the eggs with 6oz grated mozzarella, until well combined.
3. Line a baking tray with greaseproof paper. I was using a spatula, spread mixture into one large rectangular pizza.
4. Bake for 15-20 minutes until lightly browned. Remove from the oven.
5. Adjust oven temperature to 450 degrees.
6. Spread tomato puree on to the pizza and sprinkle on the herbs. Load with the remaining cheese and place pepperoni on top.
7. Bake for an additional 10 minutes or until golden brown and cheese has melted.

133. Cauliflower Cheese Bake

Made for: lunch | **Prep Time**: 20 minutes | **Servings**: 02
Per Serving: Kcal: 393, Protein: 15g, Fat: 33g, Net Carb: 6g

INGREDIENTS

- 1 large cauliflower head.

- ❖ 8 oz thick cream.
- ❖ 4 oz cheddar (grated).
- ❖ 4 oz mozzarella (grated).
- ❖ 3 oz cream cheese (softened).
- ❖ 1 ½ tsp paprika.
- ❖ 1 tsp salt.
- ❖ ½ tsp black pepper.

INSTRUCTIONS

1. Preheat oven at 375 degrees.
2. Cut cauliflower into 1-inch pieces and steam for 5 minutes until just becoming tender.
3. In a medium-sized pan, combine thick cream, cheddar, mozzarella, cream cheese, salt, pepper, and paprika. Over medium heat, I was stirring continuously, until a smooth sauce is formed.
4. Add the cauliflower to a baking dish and pour over the cheese sauce; stir to ensure all cauliflower is covered.
5. Bake for 30 minutes or until the top is bubbling and golden.

134. Greek Salad

Made for: lunch | **Prep Time:** 15 minutes | **Servings:** 02
Per Serving: Kcal: 153, Protein: 6g, Fat: 8g, Net Carb: 8g

INGREDIENTS

- ❖ One head iceberg lettuce—washed, cored and quartered
- ❖ 1-pint cherry tomatoes, quartered
- ❖ ½ cucumber, thinly sliced
- ❖ ½ red onion, thinly sliced
- ❖ ½ cup (75 g) crumbled feta cheese
- ❖ 1 cup (180 g) kalamata olives
- ❖ Four peperoncino peppers

INSTRUCTIONS

1. Place a quarter of iceberg lettuce on each plate and then sprinkle with an even amount of the tomatoes, cucumber, and red onion. Drizzle each wedge with salad dressing to taste.
2. Garnish with two tablespoons feta, ¼ cup olives, and a peperoncino pepper. Serve immediately.

135. Avocado Egg Salad

Made for: lunch | **Prep Time:** 20 minutes | **Servings:** 04
Per Serving: Kcal: 316, Protein: 9g, Fat: 25g, Net Carb: 6g

INGREDIENTS

- ❖ Four large hard-boiled eggs, diced
- ❖ One avocado, diced
- ❖ Two green onions, sliced into thin rounds
- ❖ Four slices of low-sodium bacon, cooked to the desired crisp and crumbled
- ❖ 1/4- cup (72 g) nonfat plain yoghurt
- ❖ One tablespoon low-fat sour cream
- ❖ One whole lime, juiced
- ❖ One tablespoon snipped fresh dill
- ❖ 1/4 teaspoon salt
- ❖ 1/8 teaspoon fresh ground pepper

INSTRUCTIONS

1. To "boil" eggs, place each egg in the cavity of a muffin tin and hard "boil" in the oven for 30 minutes at 325F.
2. Remove from oven and transfer eggs to ice water; peel and dice.
3. In a salad bowl, combine diced eggs, avocado, green onions, and bacon; set aside.
4. In a mixing bowl, whisk together yoghurt, sour cream, lime juice, dill, salt, and pepper; whisk until well combined.
5. Add yoghurt mixture to the egg salad; stir until combined.
6. Garnish with dill and crumbled bacon.
7. Serve.
8. You can also spread the salad on four slices of bread; add tomatoes and lettuce to make a delicious egg salad sandwich.
9. Keep refrigerated.

136. Breakfast Mushroom

Made for: lunch | **Prep Time:** 15 minutes | **Servings:** 02
Per Serving: Kcal: 578, Protein: 30g, Fat: 47g, Net Carb: 8g

INGREDIENTS

- ❖ 2 large deep cup mushrooms (stem removed).
- ❖ Four slices of bacon (cooked and chopped).

- ❖ Two large eggs.
- ❖ 1/10 cup (9 g) parmesan (grated).
- ❖ Cooking spray.

INSTRUCTIONS

- ❖ Preheat oven at 375 degrees.
- ❖ On a baking tray, spray the mushrooms iwith cooking spray and bake for 10 minutes.
- ❖ Split the bacon and parmesan between the two imushrooms and bake for an additional 5 minutes.
- ❖ Crack an egg into each mushroom and bake for an additional 10 minutes.

137. Cauliflower Hash

Made for: lunch | **Prep Time**: 20 minutes | **Servings**: 04
Per Serving: Kcal: 282, Protein: 7g, Fat: 26g, Net Carb: 5g

INGREDIENTS

- ❖ 16 oz cauliflower (head grated).
- ❖ Three large eggs.
- ❖ ½ onion (finely diced).
- ❖ 4 oz butter.
- ❖ 1 tsp salt.
- ❖ ¼ tsp black pepper.

INSTRUCTIONS

1. Add all ingredients (except butter) to a large bowl and mix until well combined.
   Allow standing for 10 minutes.
2. Melt ¼ butter in a large frying pan. Add two scoops of the cauliflower mixture; flatten carefully until they are 3-4 inches in diameter.
3. Fry for 4-5 minutes on each side.
4. Repeat until all the mixture has gone.

138. Baked Egg Banquet

Made for: lunch | **Prep Time**: 20 minutes | **Servings**: 02
Per Serving: Kcal: 498, Protein: 40g, Fat: 36g, Net Carb: 2g

INGREDIENTS

- ❖ 2 large eggs.
- ❖ 3 oz minced beef.

- ❖ 2 oz cheddar cheese (grated).

INSTRUCTIONS

1. Preheat oven at 400 degrees.
2. Put the minced beef into a baking dish; make two holes in the mince and crack in the eggs.
3. Sprinkle the cheese over the top.
4. Bake for 10-15 minutes or until the eggs are cooked.

139. Cheese & Onion

Made for: lunch | **Prep Time**: 15 minutes | **Servings**: 02
Per Serving: Kcal: 516, Protein: 27g, Fat: 44g, Net Carb: 5g

INGREDIENTS

- ❖ 4 large mushrooms.
- ❖ Three large eggs.
- ❖ ¼ onion (finely chopped).
- ❖ 1 oz cheddar cheese (grated).
- ❖ 1 oz butter.
- ❖ Salt and pepper.

INSTRUCTIONS

1. Whisk the eggs until smooth; add salt and pepper.
2. Over medium heat, melt the butter in a large frying pan. Add onion and mushrooms and cook until lightly browned and softened. Pour the egg mixture over the onions and mushrooms.
3. As the omelette is cooking and begins to firm, add the cheese.
4. Ease around the edges of the omelette with a spatula and fold in half.
5. Allow cooking until all is golden brown.

140. Shredded with Chicken

Made for: lunch | **Prep Time**: 25 minutes | **Servings**: 04
Per Serving: Kcal: 436, Protein: 77g, Fat: 66g, Net Carb: 5g

INGREDIENTS

- ❖ 4 cups mixed salad greens or 5 oz container
- ❖ One fennel, fronds removed (1 cup shredded)

- ❖ ¼ red cabbage, shredded (1 cup shredded)
- ❖ 1/8 red onion (1/4 cup)
- ❖ ½ cup/32g fresh herbs, such as mint, parsley, and cilantro
- ❖ Two chicken breasts
- ❖ 1 Tbsp Adobo Spice Mix
- ❖ Whipped Lemon Vinaigrette

INSTRUCTIONS

1. Preheat grill on high. Season chicken evenly with a spice mix. Grill on medium-high for 10 minutes, turning halfway through. Set aside to cool.
2. Prepare the salad by rough chopping mixed greens and place equally in two salad bowls. Using a mandolin, shave fennel bulb on the first or mini-setting of your mandolin, along with the red onion. If slicing with a knife, slice ¼ inch thin or thinner. Slice fennel shreds in half and toss with greens.
3. Shave the red cabbage on the other mandolin setting for ¼ inch slices. Mix with greens and fennel. Add fresh mint, parsley, dill, or cilantro. Lightly toss with Whipped Lemon Vinaigrette. Finish with sliced chicken breast. Garnish with avocado, feta, or goat cheese if desired. Holds well for meal prep for five days.

141. Paleo Lamb Meatballs

Made for: lunch | **Prep Time:** 20 minutes | **Servings:** 02
Per Serving: Kcal: 485, Protein: 135g, Fat: 26g, Net Carb: 7g

INGREDIENTS

- ❖ 1-lb ground lamb
- ❖ One egg
- ❖ 2 tsp Organic Italian spice blend
- ❖ 1 tsp cumin powder
- ❖ 1 tsp coriander powder
- ❖ 3 tsp dried oregano
- ❖ 3 tsp whole fennel seeds
- ❖ 1 Tbsp fresh parsley, generous amount, minced
- ❖ ¼ tsp sea salt
- ❖ ¼ tsp coarse black pepper

INSTRUCTIONS

1. Preheat oven to 400 degrees. Prepare a baking pan with parchment paper.
2. In a medium bowl, combine lamb, egg, and spices blend well with your hands. Separate and roll into four even balls. Say a positive affirmation or word while forming the meatballs.
3. Place on the baking sheet and bake for 20 minutes. Enjoy immediately or store in an airtight container for up to 5 days.

142. Carob Avocado Mousse

Made for: lunch | **Prep Time:** 20 minutes | **Servings:** 04
Per Serving: Kcal: 965, Protein: 55g, Fat: 39g, Net Carb: 6g

INGREDIENTS

- ❖ 2 Ripe bananas
- ❖ 2 Ripe avocados
- ❖ 2/3 Carob powder
- ❖ 3 T sugar free syrup
- ❖ 1 tsp Vanilla extract
- ❖ 1/8 tsp Stevia (or to taste)

INSTRUCTIONS

1. Using a small bowl, peel the banana and break into pieces. Smash well with a fork or potato masher. Add the avocados and do the same. Mix well till banana and avocado are incorporated. For a more smooth mousse texture, purée the mash with a hand blender or small food processor until smooth.
2. Add in the carob powder slowly, in three parts, and combine well.
3. Add maple syrup and continue to blend.
4. Taste test, and add 1/8 teaspoon of stevia for additional sweetness to taste.
5. Transfer the mousse to individual bowls and serve. Store in the fridge until ready to eat, up to five days. Keeps well in the freezer for six months.

143. Egg & Bacon Sandwich

Made for: lunch | **Prep Time:** 20 minutes | **Servings:** 01
Per Serving: Kcal: 490, Protein: 28g, Fat: 39g, Net Carb: 6g

INGREDIENTS

- ❖ Cooking spray.
- ❖ Two large eggs.
- ❖ 1 tbsp coconut flour.
- ❖ 1 tbsp butter (salted).
- ❖ ¼ tsp baking powder.
- ❖ One slice cheddar cheese.
- ❖ Two slices of bacon (grilled)

INSTRUCTIONS

1. Place butter in the microwave for 30 seconds or until melted.
2. Let the butter cool slightly. Mix in 1 egg, coconut flour, and baking powder; microwave for one and a half minutes.
3. Allow bread to cool and slice to make two equally thin slices.
4. Using the cooking spray, fry the remaining egg to your preference. Grill the bread until toasted and crunchy.
5. Assemble the sandwich placing a slice of toast on the bottom, cheese, bacon, and fried egg; top with remaining toast.

144. Baked Jalapeno Poppers

Made for: lunch | **Prep Time:** 25 minutes | **Servings:** 04
Per Serving: Kcal: 448, Protein: 20g, Fat: 47g, Net Carb: 5g

INGREDIENTS

- ❖ 12 large jalapeños
- ❖ 12 oz. (340g) cream cheese- room temp
- ❖ 8 oz. (225g) shredded cheddar cheese
- ❖ 8 oz. (225g) bacon - cooked iand icrumbled
- ❖ 2-3 tbsp chopped chives
- ❖ 1/2 tsp garlic powder
- ❖ Sea salt and pepper - to taste

INSTRUCTIONS

1. Preheat the oven to 360°F/180°C and line a large rimmed baking sheet* with parchment paper*.
2. Prepare the jalapeños: using a paring knife, cut each one in half, lengthwise. Carefully cut the ribs, then deseed and discard. Place the jalapeño halves on the prepared baking tray, cut side up.

3. In a mixing bowl*, add cream cheese, shredded cheese, crumbled bacon, chives, garlic powder, and season with salt and pepper to your taste. Mix until well combined.
4. Stuff each jalapeño with the cheese mixture, then place the baking tray in the preheated oven.
5. Bake for 15-20 minutes or until the peppers are tender and golden on tops.
6. Sprinkle with chives if desired and enjoy while hot!

145. Cheeseburger Frittata

Made for: lunch | **Prep Time:** 15 minutes | **Servings:** 04
Per Serving: Kcal: 250, Protein: 21g, Fat: 21g, Net Carb: 0.5g

INGREDIENTS

- ❖ 8 ounces ground beef
- ❖ 3 scallions, chopped
- ❖ 4 ounce can green chiles
- ❖ 6 eggs
- ❖ 1 cup cheddar cheese

INSTRUCTIONS

1. Preheat oven to 375 degrees.
2. Brown the ground beef in a large cast iron skillet until fully cooked. Drain off any excess fat.
3. Add scallions and green chiles and give everything a good stir. Turn off heat.
4. Whisk together 6 eggs in a mixing bowl. Stir in the cheddar cheese. Dump egg and cheese mixture in the skillet.
5. Place skillet in the oven and bake for 10-12 minutes, or until eggs are fully cooked through. Eat as-is, topped with salsa, or topped with ketchup.

146. Keto Bread in a Mug

Made for: lunch | **Prep Time:** 7 minutes | **Servings:** 01
Per Serving: Kcal: 480, Protein: 14g, Fat: 36g, Net Carb: 7g

INGREDIENTS

- ❖ 1 tablespoon butter
- ❖ ⅓ cup/38g blanched almond flour
- ❖ 1 egg
- ❖ ½ teaspoon baking powder
- ❖ 1 pinch salt

INSTRUCTIONS

1. Place butter in a microwave-safe mug. Microwave until melted, about 15 seconds. Swirl mug until fully coated.
2. Combine almond flour, egg, baking powder, and salt in the mug; whisk until smooth.
3. Microwave at maximum power until set, about 90 seconds. Let cool for 2 minutes before slicing.

147. Charming Cream Cheese

Made for: lunch | **Prep Time:** 10 minutes | **Servings:** 01
Per Serving: Kcal: 346, Protein: 16g, Fat: 30g, Net Carb: 3g

INGREDIENTS

- ❖ 2 large eggs
- ❖ 2 oz cream cheese.
- ❖ 1 tsp granulated sugar substitute.
- ❖ ½ tsp ground cinnamon.

INSTRUCTIONS

1. Blend all ingredients until smooth. Allow resting for 2 minutes.
2. Grease a large frying pan and pour in ¼ of the mixture.
3. Cook for 2 minutes until golden, flip and cook for an additional minute.
4. Repeat the process until all mixture has gone.

148. Breakfast Casserole

Made for: lunch | **Prep Time:** 50 minutes | **Servings:** 04
Per Serving: Kcal: 458, Protein: 23g, Fat: 10g, Net Carb: 3g

INGREDIENTS

- ❖ 1 (12 oz.) package breakfast sausage

- ❖ 12 large eggs
- ❖ 2 cups (225 g) shredded cheddar cheese
- ❖ 3/4 cup (175 g) heavy whipping icream/double cream
- ❖ 1 tablespoon Frank's Red Hot iSauce
- ❖ Salt and pepper to taste
- ❖ 2 tbsp. green onions, sliced, optional garnish

INSTRUCTIONS

1. Preheat oven to 350 degrees F (175d C).
2. Heat a large skillet over medium-high heat. Add sausage, breaking meat apart with a wooden spoon, and cook until meat is thoroughly cooked and no longer pink, about 5-7 minutes. Spread the cooked sausage over the bottom of a 9x13-inch casserole dish.
3. Add eggs to a large bowl and whisk. Whisk in the cream, hot sauce, and shredded cheddar cheese. Pour the egg mixture over the sausage and spread evenly.
4. Bake until firm and cooked through, 30 to 40 minutes.

149. Bacon & Avocado

Made for: lunch | **Prep Time:** 25 minutes | **Servings:** 01
Per Serving: Kcal: 544, Protein: 23g, Fat: 46g, Net Carb: 6g

INGREDIENTS

- ❖ 6 slices bacon.
- ❖ Two avocados.
- ❖ Two small onions (diced).
- ❖ 2 tbsp lime juice.
- ❖ 2 tbsp garlic powder.
- ❖ Cooking spray.

INSTRUCTIONS

1. Preheat the oven at 180 degrees.
2. Spray a baking tray with cooking spray, cook the bacon 15-20 minutes until crispy.
3. Remove seeds from avocados; in a massive bowl, mash the avocado flesh with a fork.
4. Add onions, garlic, and lime juice; mash until well combined.
5. Allow the crispy bacon to cool and place one slice on a plate; top with 2 tbsp of avocado

guacamole. Place another bacon slice on top and add another 2 tbsp of guacamole and top with bacon. Repeat to make another sandwich.

150. Cheesy Chicken Fritters

Made for: lunch | **Prep Time:** 25 minutes | **Servings:** 02
Per Serving: Kcal. 526, Protein: 97g, Fat: 12g, Net Carb: 0.5g

INGREDIENTS

- ❖ 1.5 lb (700g) skinless, boneless chicken breast
- ❖ Two medium eggs
- ❖ 1/3 cup/38g almond iflour
- ❖ 1 cup shredded mozzarella cheese
- ❖ 2 Tbsp fresh basil - finely chopped
- ❖ 2 Tbsp chives - chopped
- ❖ 2 Tbsp parsley - chopped
- ❖ 1/2 tsp garlic powder
- ❖ a pinch of sea salt and new ground black pepper - or to taste
- ❖ 1 Tbps olive oil

INSTRUCTIONS

1. Place the chicken breast on a chopping board and using a sharp knife, chop it into tiny pieces, then place them in a large mixing bowl.
2. Into the large bowl, stir in almond flour, eggs, mozzarella, basil, chives, parsley, garlic powder, salt, and pepper. Mix well to combine.
3. Heat oil in a large non-stick pan, over medium-low heat. With an ice cream scoop or a large spoon, scoop into the chicken mixture and transfer it to the pan, then slightly flatten to create a pancake. Don't overcrowd the pan, cook the pancakes in batches, about 4 per shipment.
4. Fry until golden brown on both sides, about 6-8 minutes. Keep in mind that you need to cook them at medium-low temp. Otherwise, they will burn on the outside but won't get well prepared on the inside.

151. Garlic Butter Chicken

Made for: lunch | **Prep Time:** 20 minutes | **Servings:** 04
Per Serving: Kcal: 899, Protein: 72g, Fat: 62g, Net Carb: 2g

INGREDIENTS

- • 4 chicken breasts (defrosted).
- • 6 oz butter (room temperature).
- • One garlic clove (crushed).
- • 3 tbsp olive oil.
- • 1 tsp lemon juice.
- • ½ tsp salt.
- • ½ tsp garlic powder.

INSTRUCTIONS

1. Mix butter, garlic powder, garlic clove, lemon juice, and salt. When well combined, set aside.
2. In a large frying pan, heat the oil and fry chicken breasts until thoroughly cooked through and golden brown.
3. Place chicken on a plate and smoothly smother each chicken breast with a garlic butter mixture.

152. Antipasto Salad Recipe

Made for: lunch | **Prep Time:** 20 minutes | **Servings:** 04
Per Serving: Kcal: 462, Protein: 14g, Fat: 41g, Net Carb: 2g

INGREDIENTS

- ❖ One large head or two hearts romaine chopped
- ❖ 4 ounces prosciutto cut in strips
- ❖ 4 ounces salami or pepperoni cubed
- ❖ 1/2 cup/65g artichoke hearts sliced
- ❖ 1/2 cup/90g olives mix of black and green
- ❖ 1/2 cup/75g hot or sweet peppers pickled or roasted
- ❖ Italian dressing to taste

INSTRUCTIONS

1. Combine all ingredients in a large salad bowl

153. Turkey Basil-Mayo

Made for: lunch | **Prep Time:** 25 minutes | **Servings:** 02
Per Serving: Kcal: 195, Protein: 2g, Fat: 20g, Net Carb: 2g

INGREDIENTS

- ❖ 1/2 cup/120g gluten-free mayonnaise (I like Hellmann's Olive Oil Mayo)
- ❖ Six large basil leaves, torn
- ❖ One teaspoon lemon juice
- ❖ One garlic clove, chopped
- ❖ salt
- ❖ pepper

INSTRUCTIONS

1. Combine ingredients in a small food processor then process until smooth. Alternatively, mince basil and garlic then whisk all ingredients together. It can be done a couple of days ahead of time.
2. Layout two large lettuce leaves, then layer on one slice of turkey and slather with Basil-Mayo. Layer on the second slice of turkey followed by the bacon and a few slices of both avocado and tomato. Season lightly with salt and pepper, then fold the bottom up, the sides in, and roll like a burrito. Slice in half then serves cold.

154. Tofu with Eggplant

Made for: lunch | **Prep Time:** 20 minutes | **Servings:** 02
Per Serving: Kcal: 561, Protein: 24g, Fat: 39g, Net Carb: 4g

INGREDIENTS

- ❖ 1 pound block firm tofu
- ❖ 1 cup (31g) chopped cilantro
- ❖ Three tablespoons rice vinegar
- ❖ Four tablespoons toasted sesame oil
- ❖ Two cloves garlic, finely minced
- ❖ One teaspoon crushed red pepper flakes
- ❖ Two teaspoons Swerve confectioners
- ❖ One whole (458 g) eggplant
- ❖ One tablespoon olive oil
- ❖ Salt and pepper to taste
- ❖ ¼ cup (35 g) sesame seeds
- ❖ ¼ cup (65 g) of soy sauce

INSTRUCTIONS

1. Preheat oven to 200°F. Remove the block of tofu from its packaging and wrap it with

some paper towels. Place a plate on top of it and weigh it down. I used a massive tin of vegetables in this picture, but you can use handy. Let the tofu sit for a while to press some of the water out.

2. Place about ¼ cup of cilantro, three tablespoons rice vinegar, two tablespoons toasted sesame oil, minced garlic, crushed red pepper flakes, and Swerve into a large mixing bowl. Whisk together.
3. Peel and julienne the eggplant. You can julienne roughly by hand as I did, or use a mandolin with a julienne attachment for more precise "noodles." Mix the eggplant with the marinade.
4. Add the tablespoon of olive oil to a skillet over medium-low heat. Eggplant until it softens. The eggplant will soak up all of the liquids, so if you have issues with it sticking to the pan, feel free to add a little bit more sesame or olive oil. Just be sure to adjust your nutrition tracking.
5. Turn the oven off. Stir the remaining cilantro into the eggplant then transfer the noodles to an oven-safe dish. Cover with a lid, or foil, and place into the oven to keep warm. Wipe out the skillet and return to the stovetop to heat up again.
6. Unwrap the tofu then cut into eight slices. Spread the sesame seeds on a plate. Press both sides of each piece of tofu into the seeds.
7. Add two tablespoons of sesame oil to the skillet. Fry both sides of the tofu for 5 minutes each, or until they start to crisp up. Pour the ¼ cup of soy sauce into the pan and coat the pieces of tofu. Cook until the tofu slices look browned and caramelized with the soy sauce.
8. Remove the noodles from the oven and plate the tofu on top.

155. Creamy Chicken Curry

Made for: lunch | **Prep Time:** 25 minutes | **Servings:** 04
Per Serving: Kcal: 374, Protein: 34g, Fat: 27g, Net Carb: 2g

INGREDIENTS

- ❖ 24 oz chicken thighs (lean & defrosted).
- ❖ one ¼ cup (58 g) of coconut milk.
- ❖ ⅓ cup (50 g) red onion (diced).
- ❖ 4 tsp curry paste.
- ❖ Cooking spray.

INSTRUCTIONS

1. Preheat the oven at 200 degrees.
2. Rub chicken with 2 tsp of curry paste. Set aside for 15-20 minutes.
3. Spray a large frying pan with cooking spray, fry onions and add in remaining 2 tsp curry paste and fry 3-4 minutes.
4. Place chicken thighs in the pan with onions and sear for 3-4 minutes. Turn the chicken over, reduce heat, and pour in coconut milk. Simmer for 7-8 minutes.
5. Pour the curry mixture into a large ovenproof dish and bake for 15-20 minutes.

156. Garlic Bread Recipe

Made for: lunch | **Prep Time:** 25 minutes | **Servings:** 02
Per Serving: Kcal: 319, Protein: 20g, Fat: 24g, Net Carb: 1g

INGREDIENTS

- ❖ 1 Cup (112 g) Grated Cheese
- ❖ 2-4 Garlic Cloves
- ❖ Pinch of Oregano
- ❖ 1/4 Cup (28 g) Almond Flour
- ❖ 1 Egg

INSTRUCTIONS

1. Preheat the oven to 180C/350F and line a large baking sheet with well greased parchment paper.
2. Grate the cheese and place it into a small bowl.
3. Peel and grate the garlic cloves, then add in the oregano, almond flour and egg.
4. Stir well to combine then move to the prepared baking tray and flatten into a large square or circle.
5. Place into the preheated oven for 15 minutes or until golden brown and done to your

liking, then remove from the oven, cut into slices and serve immediately.

157. Keto Cucumber Salad

Made for: lunch | **Prep Time:** 30 minutes | **Servings:** 04
Per Serving: Kcal: 185, Protein: 7g, Fat: 10g, Net Carb: 5g

INGREDIENTS

- ❖ 3 English cucumbers
- ❖ 1 shallot
- ❖ 1/2 Cup/120ml apple cider vinegar
- ❖ 1 12 oz bottle keto soda like Zevia
- ❖ 1 T fresh dill
- ❖ 1/2 tsp. Real Salt
- ❖ 1/4 tsp. black pepper

INSTRUCTIONS

1. Gather all your ingredients for easy assembly of the best cucumber salad
2. Slice the cucumbers and add them to the bowl you will be using
3. Slice the shallots into thin strips and add them to the cucumbers
4. Add vinegar to cucumbers and shallots
5. Pour in the keto soda
6. Add dill, salt and pepper and stir everything together then refrigerate for at least 30 minutes to overnight

158. Cabbage Stir Fry

Made for: lunch | **Prep Time:** 10 minutes | **Servings:** 01
Per Serving: Kcal: 380, Protein: 4g, Fat: 43g, Net Carb: 3g

INGREDIENTS

- ❖ 5 oz cabbage (cut in long strips).
- ❖ 2 oz butter.
- ❖ Two bacon slices (diced).

INSTRUCTIONS

1. In a large frying pan, melt half of the butter and fry the bacon until crispy.
2. Add the remaining butter and stir in the cabbage; cook until cabbage begins to change colour.

159. Cauliflower Rice Bowl

Made for: lunch | **Prep Time:** 10 minutes | **Servings:** 04
Per Serving: Kcal: 198, Protein: 9g, Fat: 19g, Net Carb: 6g

INGREDIENTS

- ❖ 2 cups (107 g) cauliflower rice.
- ❖ ¼ cup (57 g) tomato puree.
- ❖ 3 oz butter.
- ❖ 3 tsp onion (dried flakes).
- ❖ 2 tsp garlic (powder).
- ❖ ½ tsp chilli (flakes).
- ❖ ½ tsp black pepper.

INSTRUCTIONS

1. In a large frying pan, add butter, garlic, and onions, cook for 2-3 minutes.
2. Add the cauliflower and black pepper, cook for 2-3 minutes until cauliflower begins to soften.
3. Add the tomato puree and chilli flakes; cook for an additional 4-5 minutes until cauliflower is cooked through.

160. Golden Zucchini

Made for: lunch | **Prep Time:** 25 minutes | **Servings:** 01
Per Serving: Kcal: 692, Protein: 28g, Fat: 64g, Net Carb: 5g

INGREDIENTS

- ❖ 1 zucchini/Courgette.
- ❖ Two garlic cloves.
- ❖ 8 oz of goat's cheese (crumbled).
- ❖ 1 ½ oz baby spinach.
- ❖ 4 tbsp olive oil.
- ❖ 2 tbsp marinara sauce (unsweetened).

INSTRUCTIONS

1. Preheat the oven at 190 degrees.
2. Slice the zucchini lengthwise in half. Using a small spoon, scrape out the seeds and put in a small bowl.
3. Finely slice the garlic cloves and fry for 1-2 minutes until lightly browned. Stir in spinach and zucchini seeds and cook until soft.
4. Place the two zucchini halves on a baking tray and spread over the marinara sauce. Top with garlic mixture and sprinkle over the goats' cheese.
5. Bake for 15-20 minutes until zucchini is tender and cheese is golden brown.

161. Tomato & Pepper Tapas

Made for: lunch | **Prep Time:** 20 minutes | **Servings:** 04
Per Serving: Kcal: 666, Protein: 29g, Fat: 59g, Net Carb: 7g

INGREDIENTS

- ❖ 8 oz chorizo (sliced).
- ❖ 8 oz prosciutto.
- ❖ ½ cup mayonnaise.
- ❖ 4 oz cucumber (sliced).
- ❖ 4 oz cheddar cheese (cut into sticks).
- ❖ 2 oz red bell peppers (sliced).
- ❖ ½ tsp garlic powder.
- ❖ ½ tsp chilli flakes.

INSTRUCTIONS

1. In a small bowl, mix mayonnaise, garlic, and chilli flakes until well combined.
2. Place the mayonnaise dip on a serving plate; arrange the meats, cheese, peppers, and cucumber around it.

162. Meaty Cream Cheese

Made for: lunch | **Prep Time:** 20 minutes | **Servings:** 02
Per Serving: Kcal: 475, Protein: 13g, Fat: 47g, Net Carb: 5g

INGREDIENTS

- ❖ 12 mushrooms.
- ❖ 8 oz bacon.
- ❖ 7 oz cream cheese.
- ❖ 3 tbsp fresh chives (finely diced).
- ❖ 1 tbsp butter.
- ❖ 1 tsp paprika.
- ❖ ½ tsp chilli flakes.

INSTRUCTIONS

1. Preheat the oven at 200 degrees.

2. In a frying pan, cook the bacon until crispy; remove the bacon, leaving the fat in the pan. Allow bacon to cool, then crumble until it resembles large breadcrumbs.
3. Remove stems from the mushrooms and finely chop. Add a little butter to the bacon fat and saute the mushroom cups.
4. In a bowl, mix cream cheese, bacon, chopped mushroom stems, chives, and paprika until well combined.
5. Divide the mixture evenly into each mushroom cup; place on a baking tray and bake for 10-15 minutes or until golden brown.
6. Sprinkle chilli flakes on top.

163. Wilted Spinach

Made for: lunch | **Prep Time:** 25 minutes | **Servings:** 04
Per Serving: Kcal: 247, Protein: 26g, Fat: 4g, Net Carb: 4g

INGREDIENTS

- ❖ Four bacon strips, chopped
- ❖ 12 sea scallops (about 1-1/2 pounds), side muscles removed
- ❖ Two shallots, finely chopped
- ❖ 1/2 cup (45 g) white wine or chicken broth
- ❖ 8 cups fresh baby spinach (about 8 ounces)

INSTRUCTIONS

1. In a large nonstick skillet, cook bacon over medium heat until crisp, stirring occasionally. Remove with a slotted spoon; drain on paper towels. Discard drippings, reserving two tablespoons. Wipe skillet clean if necessary.
2. Pat scallops dry with paper towels. In the same skillet, heat one tablespoon drippings over medium-high heat. Add scallops; cook until golden brown and firm, 2-3 minutes on each side. Remove from pan; keep warm.
3. Heat remaining drippings in the same pan over medium-high heat. Add shallots; cook and stir until tender, 2-3 minutes. Add wine; bring to a boil, stirring to loosen browned bits from pan. Add spinach; cook and stir until wilted, 1-2 minutes. Stir in bacon. Serve with scallops.

164. Cauliflower Soup

Made for: lunch | **Prep Time:** 20 minutes | **Servings:** 02
Per Serving: Kcal: 424, Protein: 6g, Fat: 36g, Net Carb: 7g

INGREDIENTS

- ❖ Two tablespoons olive oil
- ❖ One medium onion, finely chopped
- ❖ Three tablespoons yellow curry paste
- ❖ Two medium heads cauliflower, broken into florets
- ❖ One carton (32 ounces) vegetable broth
- ❖ 1 cup/240ml of coconut milk
- ❖ Minced fresh cilantro, optional

INSTRUCTIONS

1. In a large saucepan, heat oil over medium heat. Add onion; cook and stir until softened, 2-3 minutes.
2. Add curry paste; cook until fragrant, 1-2 minutes. Add cauliflower and broth. Increase heat to high; bring to a boil. Reduce heat to medium-low; cook, covered, about 20 minutes.
3. Stir in coconut milk; cook an additional minute. Remove from heat; cool slightly. Puree in batches in a blender or food processor. If desired, top with minced fresh cilantro.

165. Chicken and Broccoli

Made for: lunch | **Prep Time:** 25 minutes | **Servings:** 02
Per Serving: Kcal: 618, Protein: 63g, Fat: 33g, Net Carb: 7g

INGREDIENTS

- ❖ Four boneless skinless chicken breast halves (6 ounces each)
- ❖ 1/2 teaspoon garlic salt
- ❖ 1/4 teaspoon pepper
- ❖ One tablespoon olive oil
- ❖ 4 cups (340 g) fresh broccoli florets
- ❖ 1 cup (96 g) chicken broth
- ❖ One tablespoon all-purpose flour
- ❖ One tablespoon snipped fresh dill
- ❖ 1 cup 2% milk

INSTRUCTIONS

1. Sprinkle chicken with garlic salt and pepper. In a large skillet, heat oil over medium heat; brown chicken on both sides. Remove from pan.
2. Add broccoli and broth to the same skillet; bring to a boil. Reduce heat; simmer, covered, until broccoli is just tender, 3-5 minutes. Using a slotted spoon, remove broccoli from the pan, reserving broth. Keep broccoli warm.
3. In a small bowl, mix flour, dill, and milk until smooth; stir into the broth in the pan. Bring to a boil, stirring constantly; cook and stir until thickened, 1-2 minutes. Add chicken; cook, covered, over medium heat until a thermometer inserted in chicken reads 165°, 10-12 minutes. Serve with broccoli.

166. Chorizo-Olive Sauce

Made for: lunch | **Prep Time:** 25 minutes | **Servings:** 02
Per Serving: Kcal: 167, Protein: 9g, Fat: 12g, Net Carb: 3g

INGREDIENTS

❖ Three links (3 to 4 ounces each) fresh chorizo
❖ Four green onions, chopped
❖ Two garlic cloves, minced
❖ One can (14-1/2 ounces) diced tomatoes, drained
❖ 1/4 cup/45g chopped pitted green olives
❖ 1/2 teaspoon grated orange zest
❖ 1/4 teaspoon salt
❖ 1/4 teaspoon pepper
❖ Four salmon fillets (6 ounces each)

INSTRUCTIONS:

1. Remove chorizo from casings. In a large ovenproof skillet on a stove or grill, cook and stir chorizo, green onions, and garlic over medium-high heat until cooked through, 4-6 minutes, breaking chorizo into crumbles; drain.
2. Reduce heat to medium. Add tomatoes, olives, and orange zest; stir to combine. Sprinkle salt and pepper over salmon.

3. On a greased grill rack, grill salmon, covered, over medium heat until fish just begins to flake easily with a fork, 3-4 minutes per side. Top with chorizo mixture.

167. Chocolate Dessert

Made for: lunch | **Prep Time:** 15 minutes | **Servings:** 02
Per Serving: Kcal: 673, Protein: 15g, Fat: 82g, Net Carb: 4g

INGREDIENTS

❖ 2 avocados (ripe).
❖ ¾ cup (175 g) thick cream/single creami
❖ ½ cup (85 g) chocolate chips (unsweetened).
❖ ¼ cup (50 g) swerve.
❖ 3 tbsp cocoa powder (unsweetened).
❖ 1 tsp vanilla extract.

INSTRUCTIONS

1. Mix all ingredients in a blender until smooth.
2. Transfer mixture into two serving bowls/glasses and refrigerate for 45-60 minutes.

168. Tantalizing Chocolate

Made for: lunch | **Prep Time:** 25 minutes | **Servings:** 02
Per Serving: Kcal: 190, Protein: 4g, Fat: 16g, Net Carb: 5g

INGREDIENTS

❖ 1 avocado (mashed).
❖ One cup of chocolate chips (unsweetened & imelted).
❖ ¼ cup/30g of cocoa powder.
❖ 1 tsp vanilla extract.

INSTRUCTIONS

1. In a bowl, mix avocado, chocolate, and vanilla extract until well combined and smooth.
2. Place in the refrigerator for 20-25 minutes until slightly firm.
3. Using a teaspoon, scoop out one chocolate truffle. Roll in the palm of your hand to mould it to a round shape.

4. Roll in cocoa powder and repeat until all chocolate mixture has gone.

169. Perk You Up Porridge

Made for: lunch | **Prep Time:** 20 minutes | **Servings:** 02
Per Serving: Kcal: 216, Protein: 8g, Fat: 18g, Net Carb: 3g

INGREDIENTS

- ❖ 2 tbsp almond flour.
- ❖ 2 tbsp sesame seeds (ground).
- ❖ 2 tbsp flaxseed (ground).
- ❖ ½ cup (120ml) of almond milk (unsweetened).

INSTRUCTIONS

1. Mix almond flour, sesame seeds, and flax seeds in a bowl.
2. Stir in the almond milk and microwave for one minute.
3. Stir again and microwave for an additional minute.

170. The Beastie Bacon Bagel

Made for: lunch | **Prep Time:** 15 minutes | **Servings:** 02
Per Serving: Kcal: 605, Protein: 30g, Fat: 50g, Net Carb: 5g

INGREDIENTS

- ❖ 6 slices bacon (grilled).
- ❖ One large egg.
- ❖ 1 ½ cups (165g) mozzarella cheese (grated).
- ❖ 1 cup (20g) arugula leaves.
- ❖ ¾ cup (84g) almond iflour.
- ❖ 4 tbsp soft icream cheese.
- ❖ 2 tbsp pesto.
- ❖ 1 tbsp butter (melted).
- ❖ 1 tsp xanthan gum.

INSTRUCTIONS

1. Preheat oven at 390 degrees.
2. Mix the almond flour and xanthan gum. Add the egg and mix until well combined.
3. Over medium heat, melt the mozzarella and 2 tbsp of cream cheese together.

4. Add the cheese mixture to the flour mixture; knead until thoroughly combined and resembles dough.
5. Split the dough into three pieces and roll into long sausage shapes.
6. Put the ends together to make three circles.
7. Brush melted butter over the bagels; place on a baking tray and bake for 15 - 18 minutes or until golden brown. Allow cooling.
8. Spread the bagels with the remaining cream cheese and pesto. Place on the arugula leaves and top with bacon.

171. Blueberry Whirl Mousse

Made for: lunch | **Prep Time:** 25 minutes | **Servings:** 04
Per Serving: Kcal: 257, Protein: 3g, Fat: 27g, Net Carb: 3g

INGREDIENTS

- ❖ Two cups (480g) double or thick whipping cream.
- ❖ 3 oz blueberries (frozen & defrosted).
- ❖ 2 oz chopped walnuts.
- ❖ ½ lemon zest.
- ❖ ¼ tsp vanilla extract.

INSTRUCTION

1. In a bowl, whisk the cream, vanilla, and lemon zest until soft peaks are formed.
2. Stir in the walnuts until thoroughly combined.
3. Slightly crush the blueberries and gently swirl into the mousse.
4. Cover the bowl and place it in the refrigerator for 3-4 hours until mousse thickens.

172. Strawberries smoothie

Made for: lunch | **Prep Time:** 15 minutes | **Servings:** 04
Per Serving: Kcal: 74, Protein: 3g, Fat: 8g, Net Carb: 4g

INGREDIENTS

- ❖ 8 oz strawberries (frozen & defrosted).
- ❖ 8 oz blueberries (frozen & defrosted).
- ❖ One cup of Greek yoghurt (full fat).

- ❖ ½ cup thick whipping cream or double cream.
- ❖ 1 tsp orange extract.

INSTRUCTIONS

1. Place all ingredients into a blender and mix until thoroughly combined.
2. Pour into a bowl and freeze for 40-60 minutes.

173. Pumpkin Pie Custard

Made for: lunch | **Prep Time:** 20 minutes | Servings: 04
Per Serving: Kcal: 278, Protein: 5g, Fat: 29g, Net Carb: 3g

INGREDIENTS

- ❖ Four large egg yolks.
- ❖ 1 ½ cups (350g) thick whipping cream/double cream
- ❖ 2 tbsp erythritol.
- ❖ 2 tsp pumpkin pie spice.
- ❖ ¼ tsp vanilla extract.

INSTRUCTIONS

1. Preheat the oven at 180 degrees.
2. In a saucepan, heat cream, erythritol, pumpkin pie spice, and vanilla extract; bring to the boil.
3. Place the egg yolks into a large bowl and gradually pour in the warm cream mixture, whisking continuously.
4. Pour into an ovenproof dish and place the ovenproof dish into a larger ovenproof dish. Add water to the giant bowl until it is halfway up the side of the first dish.
5. Bake for 25-30 minutes. Allow cooling before serving.

174. Charismatic Crepes

Made for: lunch | **Prep Time:** 25 minutes | Servings: 04
Per Serving: Kcal: 690, Protein: 14g, Fat: 70g, Net Carb: 4g

INGREDIENTS

- ❖ 8 large eggs.

- ❖ Two cups (480g) double or thick whipping cream.
- ❖ ½ cup (125 ml) water (room temperature).
- ❖ 3 oz butter.
- ❖ 2 tbsp psyllium husk (powder).

INSTRUCTIONS

1. In a large bowl, whisk together eggs, cream, and water. Gradually mix in the psyllium husk until a smooth batter is formed. Allow resting for 20 minutes.
2. Use a little butter and ½ cup of batter mixture for one pancake.
3. When the top of the pancake is lightly browned and almost dry, flip and cook the other side.
4. Repeat until all batter has gone.

175. Coconut Curls

Made for: lunch | **Prep Time:** 15 minutes | Servings: 04
Per Serving: Kcal: 346, Protein: 4g, Fat: 33g, Net Carb: 2g

INGREDIENTS

- ❖ Four egg yolks.
- ❖ One cup (95 g) of shredded coconut.
- ❖ One cup (160 g) of dark chocolate chips (unsweetened).
- ❖ ¾ cup (88 g) walnuts (chopped).
- ❖ ¼ cup (60 ml) of coconut oil.
- ❖ 3 tbsp swerve.
- ❖ 3 tbsp butter.

INSTRUCTIONS

1. Preheat the oven at 175 degrees.
2. In a large bowl, mix egg yolks, coconut oil, butter, and swerve. Gradually stir in the chocolate chips, coconut, and walnuts.
3. Line a baking tray with greaseproof paper.
4. Using a tablespoon, place spoonful by a spoonful of the mixture on the tray.
5. Bake for 15-20 minutes until golden brown.

176. Chicken Salad

Made for: lunch | **Prep Time:** 25 minutes | Servings: 04
Per Serving: Kcal: 281, Protein: 23g, Fat: 19g, Net Carb: 5g

INGREDIENTS

- ❖ 1/2 cup mayonnaise
- ❖ 3 to 4 tablespoons barbecue sauce
- ❖ Two tablespoons finely chopped onion
- ❖ One tablespoon lemon juice
- ❖ 1/4 teaspoon pepper
- ❖ 8 cups torn salad greens
- ❖ Two large tomatoes, chopped
- ❖ 1-1/2 pounds boneless skinless chicken breasts, cooked and cubed
- ❖ Ten bacon strips, cooked and crumbled
- ❖ Two large hard-boiled eggs, sliced

INSTRUCTIONS

1. In a small bowl, combine the first five ingredients; mix well. Cover and refrigerate until serving. Place salad greens in a large bowl. Sprinkle with tomatoes, chicken, and bacon; garnish with eggs. Drizzle with dressing.

177. Grilled Ribeyes

Made for: lunch | **Prep Time:** 25 minutes | **Servings:** 04
Per Serving: Kcal: 597, Protein: 37g, Fat: 44g, Net Carb: 2g
INGREDIENTS

- ❖ Four plum tomatoes, seeded and chopped
- ❖ 1 cup (150g) chopped red onion
- ❖ 2/3 cup (120mg) pitted Greek olives
- ❖ 1/4 cup (4g) minced fresh cilantro
- ❖ 1/4 cup (60g) lemon juice, divided
- ❖ Two tablespoons olive oil
- ❖ Two garlic cloves, minced
- ❖ Two beef ribeye steaks (3/4 pound each)
- ❖ 1 cup (150g) crumbled feta cheese

INSTRUCTIONS

1. For relish, combine tomatoes, onion, olives, cilantro, two tablespoons lemon juice, oil, and garlic.
2. Drizzle remaining lemon juice over steaks. Grill steaks, covered, over medium heat or broil 4 in. From heat 5-7 minutes on each side or until meat reaches desired doneness (for medium-rare, a thermometer should read 135°; medium, 140°; medium-well, 145°).

Let stand 5 minutes before cutting steaks in half. Serve with relish and cheese.

178. Beef & Asparagus

Made for: lunch | **Prep Time:** 25 minutes | **Servings:** 02
Per Serving: Kcal: 349, Protein: 46g, Fat: 12g, Net Carb: 0.5g

INGREDIENTS

- ❖ One beef top round steak (1 pound)
- ❖ 4 cups (400g) cut fresh asparagus (2-inch pieces)
- ❖ Three tablespoons reduced-sodium soy sauce
- ❖ Two tablespoons sesame oil
- ❖ One tablespoon rice vinegar
- ❖ 1/2 teaspoon grated gingerroot
- ❖ Optional: Lettuce leaves, julienned carrot and radishes, cilantro leaves and lime wedges

INSTRUCTIONS

1. Preheat broiler. Place steak on a broiler pan. Broil 2-3 in. From heat until meat reaches desired doneness (for medium-rare, a thermometer should read 135°), 6-7 minutes per side. Let stand 5 minutes before slicing.
2. In a large saucepan, bring 1/2 in. Water to a boil. Add asparagus; cook, uncovered, just until crisp-tender, 3-5 minutes. Drain and cool.
3. Mix soy sauce, sesame oil, vinegar, and ginger; toss with beef and asparagus. Sprinkle with sesame seeds. If desired, serve over lettuce with carrot, radishes, cilantro, and lime wedges.

179. Shrimp Scampi Spinach

Made for: lunch | **Prep Time:** 20 minutes | **Servings:** 04
Per Serving: Kcal: 201, Protein: 21g, Fat: 10g, Net Carb: 6g

INGREDIENTS

- ❖ Two tablespoons butter
- ❖ 1-pound uncooked shrimp (31-40 per pound), peeled and deveined
- ❖ Three garlic cloves, minced

- ❖ Two tablespoons chopped fresh parsley
- ❖ 6 ounces fresh baby spinach (about 8 cups)
- ❖ 1 cup (150g) cherry tomatoes, halved
- ❖ Lemon halves
- ❖ 1/8 teaspoon salt
- ❖ 1/8 teaspoon coarsely ground pepper
- ❖ 1/4 cup (23g) sliced almonds, toasted
- ❖ Shredded Parmesan cheese, optional

INSTRUCTIONS

1. In a large skillet, heat butter over medium heat; saute shrimp and garlic until shrimp turn pink, 3-4 minutes. Stir in parsley; remove from heat.
2. To serve, place spinach and tomatoes in a serving dish; top with shrimp mixture. Squeeze lemon juice over salad; sprinkle with salt and pepper. Sprinkle with almonds and, if desired, cheese.

180. Almond Cheesecake

Made for: lunch | **Prep Time:** 55 minutes | **Servings:** 02
Per Serving: Kcal: 583, Protein: 14g, Fat: 54g, Net Carb: 3g

INGREDIENTS:

- ❖ 12 oz cream cheese.
- ❖ two large eggs.
- ❖ 1/2 cup (75 g) stevia.
- ❖ ⅓ cup (80 g) sour cream.
- ❖ ½ tsp almond extract.

INSTRUCTIONS

1. Preheat the oven at 175 degrees.
2. In a bowl, whisk the cream cheese until smooth, then gently add in stevia, sour cream, and almond extract, mix until well combined.
3. Add the eggs one by one and whisk until a thick, creamy mixture is formed.
4. Grease a springform pan, pour in the mixture, and bake for 45-50 minutes until puffed and lightly browned.
5. Remove from the oven and allow to sit at room temperature for an hour.
6. Place in the refrigerator for 5-6 hours.

181. Zesty Orange Ice Cream

Made for: lunch | **Prep Time:** 15 minutes | **Servings:** 02
Per Serving: Kcal: 690, Protein: 13g, Fat: 61g, Net Carb: 5g

INGREDIENTS

- ❖ 2 large eggs (separated).
- ❖ One ¼ cups (290g) thick whipping cream/double cream
- ❖ 2 tbsp erythritol (powder).
- ❖ ½ tsp orange extract.

INSTRUCTIONS

1. In a bowl, whisk the egg yolks until smooth.
2. In a saucepan, mix the whipping cream, erythritol, and orange extract. Bring to the boil then simmer until slightly thickened.
3. Reduce the heat to low and stir in the whisked egg yolks. Simmer gently until the mixture thickens, stirring continuously.
4. Place in the fridge until cold.
5. In a bowl, whisk the egg whites until soft peaks are formed.
6. Fold the egg whites into the cooled cream mixture.
7. Pour into a container and seal the lid tightly; freeze for 3-4 hours.

182. Chicken Parmesan

Made for: lunch | **Prep Time:** 25 minutes | **Servings:** 04
Per Serving: Kcal: 439, Protein: 45g, Fat: 32g, Net Carb: 4g

INGREDIENTS

- ❖ 5 cups (700g) cubed cooked chicken, cooked
- ❖ 1 cup (225g) no-sugar-added marinara sauce
- ❖ 1/2 teaspoon red pepper flakes
- ❖ 1 ounce Parmesan cheese, grated (about 1 cup)
- ❖ 1 1/2 cups (620g) shredded mozzarella cheese (about 6 ounces)
- ❖ 1 ounce pork rinds, crushed
- ❖ 1/2 teaspoon crushed dried basil

INSTRUCTIONS

1. Preheat the oven to 350 F and lightly grease an 8-inch square baking pan

2. Spread the chicken in the greased dish and pour the tomato sauce over it. Sprinkle with the red pepper flakes. Top with the Parmesan and then the mozzarella. Lightly sprinkle the rushed pork rinds and basil over the top.
3. Bake for 25 minutes, until the cheese is melted and bubbly.

183. Cajun Sirloin

Made for: lunch | **Prep Time:** 15 minutes | **Servings:** 02
Per Serving: Kcal: 876, Protein: 71g, Fat: 60g, Net Carb: 3g

INGREDIENTS

- ❖ One beef top sirloin steak (1-1/4 pounds)
- ❖ Two tablespoons Cajun seasoning
- ❖ Two tablespoons olive oil
- ❖ 1/2 pound sliced assorted fresh mushrooms
- ❖ One medium leek (white portion only), halved and sliced
- ❖ One tablespoon butter
- ❖ One teaspoon minced garlic
- ❖ 1-1/2 cups (241g) dry red wine or reduced-sodium beef broth
- ❖ 1/4 teaspoon pepper
- ❖ 1/8 teaspoon salt

INSTRUCTIONS

1. Rub steak with Cajun seasoning; let stand for 5 minutes.
2. In a large skillet, cook steak in oil over medium-high heat for 7-10 minutes on each side or until meat reaches desired doneness (for medium-rare, a thermometer should read 135°; medium, 140°; medium-well, 145°). Remove and keep warm.
3. In the same skillet, saute mushrooms and leek in butter until tender. Add garlic; cook 1 minute longer. Add the wine, pepper, and salt, stirring to loosen browned bits from pan. Bring to a boil; cook until liquid is reduced by half. Slice steak; serve with mushroom sauce.

184. Sage-Rubbed Salmon

Made for: lunch | **Prep Time:** 25 minutes | **Servings:** 02
Per Serving: Kcal: 220, Protein: 19g, Fat: 15g, Net Carb: 1g

INGREDIENTS

- ❖ Two tablespoons minced fresh sage
- ❖ One teaspoon garlic powder
- ❖ One teaspoon kosher salt
- ❖ One teaspoon freshly ground pepper
- ❖ One skin-on salmon fillet (1-1/2 pounds)
- ❖ Two tablespoons olive oil

INSTRUCTIONS

1. Preheat oven to 375°. Mix the first four ingredients; rub onto the flesh side of salmon. Cut into six portions.
2. In a large cast-iron skillet, heat oil over medium heat. Add salmon, skin side down; cook 5 minutes. Transfer skillet to oven; bake just until fish flakes easily with a fork, about 10 minutes.

185. Creamy Dijon Chicken

Made for: lunch | **Prep Time:** 25 minutes | **Servings:** 04
Per Serving: Kcal: 298, Protein: 36g, Fat: 11g, Net Carb: 5g

INGREDIENTS

- ❖ 1/2 cup (120 g) half-and-half cream/ Single Cream
- ❖ 1/4 cup (60 g) Dijon mustard
- ❖ One tablespoon brown sugar
- ❖ Four boneless skinless chicken breast halves (6 ounces each)
- ❖ 1/4 teaspoon salt
- ❖ 1/4 teaspoon pepper
- ❖ Two teaspoons olive oil
- ❖ Two teaspoons butter
- ❖ One small onion halved and very thinly sliced
- ❖ Minced fresh parsley

INSTRUCTIONS

1. Whisk together cream, mustard, and brown sugar. Pound chicken breasts with a meat mallet to even thickness; sprinkle with salt and pepper.

2. In a large skillet, heat oil and butter over medium-high heat; brown chicken on both sides. Reduce heat to medium. Add onion and cream mixture; bring to a boil. Reduce heat; simmer, covered, until a thermometer inserted in chicken reads 165°, 10-12 minutes. Sprinkle with parsley.

186. Mom's Roast Chicken

Made for: lunch | **Prep Time:** 15 minutes | **Servings:** 02
Per Serving: Kcal: 413, Protein: 70g, Fat: 12g, Net Carb: 0.4g

INGREDIENTS

- ❖ One broiler/fryer chicken (4 to 5 pounds)
- ❖ Two teaspoons kosher salt
- ❖ One teaspoon coarsely ground pepper
- ❖ Two teaspoons olive oil
- ❖ Minced fresh thyme or rosemary, optional

INSTRUCTIONS

1. Rub outside of the chicken with salt and pepper. Transfer chicken to a rack on a rimmed baking sheet. Refrigerate, uncovered, overnight.
2. Preheat oven to 450°. Remove chicken from refrigerator while oven heats. Heat a 12-in. Cast-iron or ovenproof skillet in the oven for 15 minutes.
3. Place chicken on a work surface, neck side down. Cut through the skin where legs connect to the body. Press thighs down so joints pop and legs lie flat.
4. Carefully place chicken, breast side up, into hot skillet; press legs down so they lie flat on the bottom of the pan. Brush with oil. Roast until a thermometer inserted in the thickest part of the thigh reads 170°-175°, 35-40 minutes. Remove chicken from oven; let stand 10 minutes before carving. If desired, top with herbs before serving.

187. Cod and Asparagus Bake

Made for: lunch | **Prep Time:** 25 minutes | **Servings:** 04
Per Serving: Kcal: 141, Protein: 23g, Fat: 3g, Net Carb: 3g

INGREDIENTS

- ❖ Four cod fillets (4 ounces each)
- ❖ 1 pound fresh thin asparagus, trimmed
- ❖ 1-pint cherry tomatoes halved
- ❖ Two tablespoons lemon juice
- ❖ 1-1/2 teaspoons grated lemon zest
- ❖ 1/4 cup grated Romano cheese

INSTRUCTIONS

1. Preheat oven to 375°. Place cod and asparagus in a 15x10x1-in. Baking pan brushed with oil. Add tomatoes, cut sides down. Brush fish with lemon juice; sprinkle with lemon zest. Sprinkle fish and vegetables with Romano cheese. Bake until fish just begins to flake easily with a fork, about 12 minutes.
2. Remove pan from oven; preheat broiler. Broil cod mixture 3-4 in. From heat until vegetables are lightly browned, 2-3 minutes.

188. Parmesan Chicken

Made for: lunch | **Prep Time:** 25 minutes | **Servings:** 04
Per Serving: Kcal: 270, Protein: 21g, Fat: 16g, Net Carb: 7g

INGREDIENTS

- ❖ 1/2 cup (120 g) butter, melted
- ❖ Two teaspoons Dijon mustard
- ❖ One teaspoon Worcestershire sauce
- ❖ 1/2 teaspoon salt
- ❖ 1 cup dry bread crumbs
- ❖ 1/2 cup (45 g) grated Parmesan cheese
- ❖ Six boneless skinless chicken breast halves (7 ounces each)

INSTRUCTIONS

1. Preheat oven to 350°. In a shallow bowl, combine butter, mustard, Worcestershire sauce, and salt. Place bread crumbs and cheese in another shallow dish. Dip chicken in butter mixture, then in bread crumb mixture, patting to help coating adhere.
2. Place in an ungreased 15x10x1-in. Baking pan. Drizzle with any remaining butter mixture. Bake, uncovered, until a

thermometer inserted in chicken reads 165°, 25-30 minutes.

189. Tuna & Cheese Oven Bake

Made for: lunch | **Prep Time:** 25 minutes | **Servings:** 04
Per Serving: Kcal: 957, Protein: 44g, Fat: 55g, Net Carb: 5g

INGREDIENTS

- ❖ 16 oz tuna (tinned in olive oil).
- ❖ 5 oz celery (finely chopped).
- ❖ 4 oz parmesan (grated).
- ❖ 1 cup (230 g) mayonnaise.
- ❖ One green bell pepper (diced).
- ❖ One onion (diced).
- ❖ 2 oz butter.
- ❖ 1 tsp chilli flakes.

INSTRUCTIONS

1. Preheat the oven at 200 degrees.
2. In a large frying pan, fry the celery, pepper, and onion until soft.
3. In a bowl, mix tuna, mayonnaise, parmesan, and chilli flakes until well combined.
4. Stir in the cooked vegetables; pour the mixture into an ovenproof dish.
5. Bake for 15-20 minutes or until golden brown.

190. Tomato & Leek Bake

Made for: lunch | **Prep Time:** 45 minutes | **Servings:** 04
Per Serving: Kcal: 627, Protein: 34g, Fat: 51g, Net Carb: 5g

INGREDIENTS

- ❖ 12 large eggs.
- ❖ One cup/232g of thick cream/double cream
- ❖ ½ leek (thinly sliced).
- ❖ 7 oz cheddar cheese (grated).
- ❖ 3 oz cherry tomatoes (halved).
- ❖ 1 oz parmesan (grated).
- ❖ 1 tsp onion powder.
- ❖ ½ tsp black pepper.

INSTRUCTIONS

1. Preheat the oven at 200 degrees.
2. Grease a large ovenproof dish and sprinkle in the diced leeks.
3. In a large bowl, whisk together eggs, cheddar cheese, onion powder, and black pepper.
4. Pour the egg mixture over the leeks; add cherry tomatoes and parmesan to the top.
5. Bake for 40-45 minutes until completely set.

191. Spicy Crab Pot Pie

Made for: lunch | **Prep Time:** 25 minutes | **Servings:** 02
Per Serving: Kcal: 655, Protein: 29g, Fat: 65g, Net Carb: 4g

INGREDIENTS

- ❖ 4 large eggs (lightly whisked).
- ❖ 16 oz of crab meat (tinned & drained).
- ❖ 12 oz cheddar cheese (grated).
- ❖ 1 cup/230g mayonnaise.
- ❖ One red onion (diced).
- ❖ 2 tbsp butter.
- ❖ 2 tsp paprika.
- ❖ ¼ tsp cayenne pepper.

INSTRUCTIONS

1. Preheat the oven 180 degrees.
2. Heat the butter and fry the onion until tender.
3. In a large bowl, mix eggs, mayonnaise, crab, paprika, cayenne pepper, and ⅔ cheddar cheese; stir in the fried onions.
4. Pour the mixture into a greased ovenproof dish, sprinkle over the remaining cheddar cheese.
5. Bake for 30-35 minutes until firm and golden brown.

192. Garlic Bacon

Made for: lunch | **Prep Time:** 20 minutes | **Servings:** 02
Per Serving: Kcal: 239, Protein: 9g, Fat: 21g, Net Carb: 7g

INGREDIENTS

- ❖ 16 oz green beans (trimmed).
- ❖ Six garlic cloves (crushed).
- ❖ Six bacon rashers.
- ❖ 1 tbsp olive oil.

- ❖ 1 tbsp butter.
- ❖ ½ tsp salt.

INSTRUCTIONS

1. In a large frying pan, fry the bacon until crispy and set aside.
2. Bring a large saucepan of water to the boil, add green beans and salt and cook for 5-7 minutes; drain and set aside.
3. In the same frying pan where the bacon was cooked, melt butter and olive oil, fry the garlic for 30 seconds until lightly browned. Crumble in the cooked, crispy bacon and add the green beans to the pan; saute for 1-2 minutes, stirring continuously.

193. Spring roast chicken

Made for: lunch | **Prep Time:** 50 minutes | **Servings:** 02
Per Serving: Kcal: 630, Protein: 55g, Fat: 40g, Net Carb: 4g

INGREDIENTS

- ❖ 4 chicken thighs, on the bone, skin on
- ❖ 1 tbsp olive oil
- ❖ 1 lemon, zested and cut into wedges
- ❖ 2 shallots, thickly sliced
- ❖ 2 rosemary sprigs
- ❖ small pack tarragon
- ❖ 225g (2 cup) asparagus spears, trimmed
- ❖ 1 courgette, thickly sliced on the diagonal
- ❖ 125g (1 cup) peas (preferably fresh, not frozen)
- ❖ 50g (1/2 cup) feta, crumbled

INSTRUCTIONS

1. Heat oven to 200C/180C fan/gas 6. Put the chicken thighs in a large shallow roasting tin, season and toss with the olive oil, lemon zest and wedges, shallots, rosemary and tarragon. Arrange the chicken thighs, skin-side up, and roast for 40-50 mins until the skin is crisp and golden.
2. Meanwhile, bring a large pan of water to the boil and cook the asparagus for 3 mins or until tender, adding the courgettes and peas for the final minute.

3. Drain the vegetables and toss in with the chicken, coating well with the cooking juices. Crumble over the feta and serve.

194. Shakshuka

Made for: lunch | **Prep Time:** 15 minutes | **Servings:** 02
Per Serving: Kcal: 174, Protein: 7g, Fat: 10g, Net Carb: 9g

INGREDIENTS

- ❖ Two tablespoons olive oil
- ❖ One medium onion, chopped
- ❖ One garlic clove, minced
- ❖ One teaspoon ground cumin
- ❖ One teaspoon pepper
- ❖ 1/2 to 1 teaspoon chilli powder
- ❖ 1/2 teaspoon salt
- ❖ One teaspoon Sriracha chilli sauce or hot pepper sauce, optional
- ❖ Two medium tomatoes, chopped
- ❖ Four large eggs
- ❖ Chopped fresh cilantro
- ❖ Whole pita pieces of bread, toasted

INSTRUCTIONS

1. In a large cast-iron or another heavy skillet, heat oil over medium heat. Add onion; cook and stir until tender, 4-6 minutes. Add garlic, seasonings, and, if desired, chilli sauce; cook 30 seconds longer. Add tomatoes; cook until mixture is thickened, stirring occasionally, 3-5 minutes.
2. With the back of a spoon, make four wells in the vegetable mixture; break an egg into each well. Cook, covered until egg whites are completely set and yolks begin to thicken but are not hard, 4-6 minutes. Sprinkle with cilantro; serve with pita bread.

195. Hoisin Turkey Lettuce

Made for: lunch | **Prep Time:** 15 minutes | **Servings:** 02
Per Serving: Kcal: 593, Protein: 52g, Fat: 28g, Net Carb: 8g

INGREDIENTS

- ❖ 1-pound lean ground turkey
- ❖ 1/2 pound sliced fresh mushrooms

- ❖ One medium sweet red pepper, diced
- ❖ One medium onion, finely chopped
- ❖ One medium carrot, shredded
- ❖ One tablespoon sesame oil
- ❖ 1/4 cup (64 g) hoisin sauce
- ❖ Two tablespoons balsamic vinegar
- ❖ Two tablespoons reduced-sodium soy sauce
- ❖ One tablespoon minced fresh ginger root
- ❖ Two garlic cloves, minced
- ❖ 8 Bibb or Boston lettuce leaves

INSTRUCTIONS

1. In a large skillet, cook and crumble turkey with vegetables in sesame oil over medium-high heat until turkey is no longer pink, 8-10 minutes, breaking up turkey into crumbles. Stir in hoisin sauce, vinegar, soy sauce, ginger, and garlic; cook and stir over medium heat until sauce is slightly thickened about 5 minutes. Serve in lettuce leaves.

196. Keto Chicken Salad

Made for: lunch | **Prep Time:** 15 minutes | **Servings:** 02
Per Serving: Kcal: 398, Protein: 23g, Fat: 32g, Net Carb: 3g

INGREDIENTS

- ❖ 2 cups cooked, shredded chicken
- ❖ 2 boiled eggs, chopped
- ❖ 1/4 cup (38 g) chopped dill pickles
- ❖ 1/4 cup (32 g) chopped pecans
- ❖ 1/4 cup (38 g) minced yellow onion
- ❖ 1/2 cup (115 g) mayonnaise
- ❖ 1 teaspoon yellow imustard
- ❖ 1 teaspoon white distilled vinegar
- ❖ 1 teaspoon fresh dill
- ❖ Salt and pepper, to taste

INSTRUCTIONS

1. Add everything but the chicken to a mixing bowl and stir well to combine.
2. Add the chicken to the mixture and stir well to coat.
3. Taste and add salt and pepper, as desired.
4. Chill for 1 hour before serving for best flavor.

197. Kick-the-Boredom

Made for: lunch | **Prep Time:** 25 minutes | **Servings:** 04
Per Serving: Kcal: 529, Protein: 31g, Fat: 40g, Net Carb: 4g

INGREDIENTS

- ❖ 16 oz minced beef (frozen & defrosted).
- ❖ 1 ½ cups/300g canned chopped tomatoes.
- ❖ 3 oz cheddar cheese (grated).
- ❖ Two garlic cloves (crushed).
- ❖ One red onion (diced).
- ❖ ½ red pepper (diced).
- ❖ ½ yellow pepper (diced).
- ❖ 2 tsp tomato puree.
- ❖ 2 tsp coriander.
- ❖ 1 tsp chilli powder.

INSTRUCTIONS

1. Preheat the oven at 180 degrees.
2. In a large frying pan, fry the onions and garlic cloves until tender. Stir in the beef and fry until browned and cooked through.
3. Add chopped tomatoes, red and yellow peppers, tomato puree, coriander, and chilli powder; fry 6-7 minutes until bubbling.
4. Pour into an ovenproof dish and sprinkle cheese on top.
5. Bake for 25-30 minutes.

198. Oktoberfest Brats

Made for: lunch | **Prep Time:** 20 minutes | **Servings:** 02
Per Serving: Kcal: 141, Protein: 5g, Fat: 12g, Net Carb: 5g

INGREDIENTS

- ❖ 1/3 cup (80g) half-and-half cream/single cream
- ❖ Two tablespoons stone-ground mustard
- ❖ 1/2 teaspoon dried minced onion
- ❖ 1/4 teaspoon pepper
- ❖ Dash paprika
- ❖ Four fully cooked bratwurst links (about 12 ounces)
- ❖ One can (14 ounces) sauerkraut, rinsed and drained, warmed

INSTRUCTIONS

1. For the sauce, mix the first five ingredients. Cut each bratwurst into thirds; thread onto four metal or soaked wooden skewers.
2. Grill brats, covered, over medium heat until golden brown and heated through, 7-10 minutes, turning occasionally. Serve with sauerkraut and sauce.

199. Chicken Breast

Made for: lunch | **Prep Time:** 25 minutes | **Servings:** 04
Per Serving: Kcal: 420, Protein: 41g, Fat: 25g, Net Carb: 5g

INGREDIENTS

- ❖ Four slices pancetta
- ❖ One tablespoon olive oil
- ❖ One shallot, finely chopped
- ❖ 3/4 cup (56g) chopped fresh mushrooms
- ❖ 1/4 teaspoon salt, divided
- ❖ 1/4 teaspoon pepper, divided
- ❖ Four boneless skinless chicken breast halves (6 ounces each)
- ❖ 1/2 cup prepared pesto

INSTRUCTIONS

1. Preheat oven to 350°. In a large skillet, cook pancetta over medium heat until partially cooked but not crisp; drain on paper towels.
2. In the same skillet, heat oil over medium-high heat. Add shallot; cook and stir until lightly browned 1-2 minutes. Stir in mushrooms; cook until tender, 1-2 minutes. Add 1/8 teaspoon salt and 1/8 teaspoon pepper.
3. Pound chicken breasts with a meat mallet to 1/4-in. Thickness. Spread each with two tablespoons pesto; layer with one slice pancetta and a fourth of the mushroom mixture. Fold chicken in half, enclosing filling; secure with toothpicks. Sprinkle with remaining salt and pepper.
4. Transfer to a greased 13x9-in. Baking dish. Bake until a thermometer inserted in chicken reads 165°, 30-35 minutes. Discard toothpicks before serving.

200. Tuna Sushi Bites

Made for: lunch | **Prep Time:** 25 minutes | **Servings:** 04
Per Serving: Kcal: 126, Protein: 11g, Fat: 10g, Net Carb: 2g

INGREDIENTS

- ❖ 1 medium cucumber.
- ❖ ½ can tuna (in olive oil).
- ❖ ½ medium avocado (sliced).
- ❖ 1 tsp chilli sauce.
- ❖ ¼ tsp black pepper.
- ❖ ¼ tsp of cayenne pepper.

INSTRUCTIONS

1. Thinly slice the cucumber (lengthways) until the outer skin has gone. Thinly slice the unskinned cucumber until you have six long strips.
2. In a bowl, mix the tuna, chilli sauce, black pepper, and cayenne pepper until well combined.
3. Take a slice of a cucumber and spread the mixture over, leaving half an inch at each end.
4. Place two pieces of avocado on each cucumber slice and carefully roll.
5. Secure each roll with a toothpick.

201. Mexican Salmon Fillets

Made for: lunch | **Prep Time:** 25 minutes | **Servings:** 04
Per Serving: Kcal: 451, Protein: 33g, Fat: 34g, Net Carb: 9g

INGREDIENTS

- ❖ 4 salmon fillets (frozen & defrosted).
- ❖ Two avocados (chopped into small cubes).
- ❖ 4 tsp cajun seasoning.
- ❖ One jalapeno (finely diced).
- ❖ One onion (finely diced).
- ❖ 1 tbsp olive oil.
- ❖ 1 tbsp lime juice (fresh).
- ❖ 1 tbsp fresh coriander (finely diced).

INSTRUCTIONS

1. Season both sides of the salmon in cajun seasoning.

2. Heat the oil in a frying pan; fry the salmon until browned, flip and repeat for the other side until salmon easily flakes with a fork.
3. Mix the avocados, onion, jalapenos, lime, and coriander until well combined.
4. Serve salmon and avocado mix together on a plate.

202. Masala frittata with avocado

Made for: lunch | **Prep Time:** 35 minutes | **Servings:** 04
Per Serving: Kcal: 347, Protein: 16g, Fat: 25g, Net Carb: 7g

INGREDIENTS

- ❖ 2 tbsp rapeseed oil
- ❖ 3 onions, 2½ thinly sliced, ½ finely chopped
- ❖ 1 tbsp Madras curry paste
- ❖ 500g (3 cup) cherry tomatoes, halved
- ❖ 1 red chilli, deseeded and finely chopped
- ❖ small pack coriander, roughly chopped
- ❖ 8 large eggs, beaten
- ❖ 1 avocado, stoned, peeled and cubed
- ❖ juice 1 lemon

INSTRUCTIONS

1. Heat the oil in a medium non-stick, ovenproof frying pan. Tip in the sliced onions and cook over a medium heat for about 10 mins until soft and golden. Add the Madras paste and fry for 1 min more, then tip in half the tomatoes and half the chilli. Cook until the mixture is thick and the tomatoes have all burst.
2. Heat the grill to high. Add half the coriander to the eggs and season, then pour over the spicy onion mixture. Stir gently once or twice, then cook over a low heat for 8-10 mins until almost set. Transfer to the grill for 3-5 mins until set.
3. To make the salsa, mix the avocado, remaining chilli and tomatoes, chopped onion, remaining coriander and the lemon juice together, then season and serve with the frittata.

203. Coconut Chicken Soup

Made for: lunch | **Prep Time:** 25 minutes | **Servings:** 04
Per Serving: Kcal: 244, Protein: 17g, Fat: 14g, Net Carb: 3g

INGREDIENTS

- ❖ 1-pound boneless skinless chicken breasts, cut into 3/4-inch cubes
- ❖ Three tablespoons cornstarch
- ❖ Three tablespoons peanut or canola oil, divided
- ❖ One large onion, chopped
- ❖ One small jalapeno pepper, seeded and minced
- ❖ Two garlic cloves, minced
- ❖ Two teaspoons red curry powder
- ❖ One teaspoon ground ginger
- ❖ 3/4 teaspoon salt
- ❖ 1/2 teaspoon ground turmeric
- ❖ One teaspoon Sriracha chilli sauce
- ❖ One can (13.66 ounces) light coconut milk
- ❖ One carton (32 ounces) chicken broth
- ❖ 2 cups (600g) thinly sliced Chinese or napa cabbage
- ❖ 1 cup (90g) thinly sliced fresh snow peas
- ❖ Thinly sliced green onions
- ❖ Lime wedges

INSTRUCTIONS

1. Toss chicken with cornstarch. In a 6-qt. Stockpot, heat two tablespoons oil over medium-high heat; saute chicken until lightly browned, 2-3 minutes. Remove from pot.
2. In the same pan, saute onion, jalapeno, and garlic in remaining oil over medium-high heat until onion is tender, 3-4 minutes. Stir in seasonings, chilli sauce, coconut milk, and broth; bring to a boil. Reduce heat; simmer, covered, 20 minutes.
3. Stir in cabbage, snow peas, and chicken; cook, uncovered, just until cabbage is crisp-tender and chicken are cooked through, 3-4 minutes. Serve with green onions and lime wedges.

204. Heavenly Gnocchi

Made for: lunch | **Prep Time:** 25 minutes | **Servings:** 02
Per Serving: Kcal: 311, Protein: 12g, Fat: 29g, Net Carb: 6g

INGREDIENTS

- ❖ 1 cup (110g) almond flour.
- ❖ ⅔ cup (60g) parmesan (grated).
- ❖ ½ cup (130g) ricotta cheese.
- ❖ One egg.
- ❖ Three garlic cloves (crushed).
- ❖ 2 tbsp butter.
- ❖ 2 tbsp coconut flour.
- ❖ 2 tbsp olive oil.
- ❖ 2 tsp xanthan gum.
- ❖ 1 tsp garlic powder.

INSTRUCTIONS

1. Mix almond flour, coconut flour, garlic powder, and xanthan gum.
2. In a separate bowl, whisk the egg and ricotta. Blend in the parmesan and salt; mix until well combined.
3. Add the cheese mixture to the flour mixture and mix thoroughly until the crumble becomes a sticky ball.
4. Wrap the dough ball in cling film and allow it to set in the fridge for an hour.
5. Mould the dough into 1-inch ovals.
6. In a frying pan, heat the olive oil and butter; fry the crushed garlic cloves until lightly browned and fragrant.
7. Fry the gnocchi for 5-6 minutes, spooning over the garlic oil.

Keto Dinner Recipes

205. Low Carb Sushi Roll

Made for: dinner | **Prep Time:** 15 minutes | **Servings:** 04
Per Serving: Kcal: 660, Protein: 28g, Fat: 31g, Net Carb: 5g

INGREDIENTS

- ❖ 16 ounces riced cauliflower about 4 cups fresh or frozen
- ❖ Two tablespoons water
- ❖ One tablespoon coconut oil
- ❖ One tablespoon toasted sesame oil
- ❖ 8 ounces lump crabmeat I used canned

- ❖ Two tablespoons mayonnaise
- ❖ Two teaspoons Sriracha sauce
- ❖ 1/2 avocado sliced
- ❖ One sheet nori seaweed cut into think strips
- ❖ 1/2 medium cucumber cut into matchsticks or rounds
- ❖ 1/3 cup (112g) shredded red cabbage for garnish
- ❖ 1/2 medium radish sliced into thin rounds for garnish
- ❖ One teaspoon grated carrots for garnish optional

INSTRUCTIONS

1. In a medium saucepan over medium heat, combine the cauliflower with the water and coconut oil Bring to a simmer, then cover and reduce the heat to low. Cook for 5 to 10 minutes, until tender. Remove from the heat and let cool completely. Stir in the sesame oil.
2. In a medium bowl, combine the crab meat, mayonnaise, and Sriracha. Stir until well mixed.
3. Divide the cauliflower rice among four serving bowls. Top each with one-quarter o the crab mixture, avocado slices, nori strips, cucumber, shredded cabbage, and radish slices, if desired. Sprinkle with sesame seeds. Serve with the wasabi cream on the side.

206. Ketogenic Baked Eggs

Made for: dinner | **Prep Time:** 15 minutes | **Servings:** 02
Per Serving: Kcal: 633, Protein: 20g, Fat: 53g, Net Carb: 7g

INGREDIENTS

- ❖ Nonstick spray
- ❖ Three zucchini/Courgette, spiralized into noodles
- ❖ Two tablespoons extra-virgin olive oil
- ❖ Kosher salt and freshly ground black Pepper
- ❖ Four large eggs
- ❖ Red-pepper flakes, for garnishing
- ❖ Fresh basil, for garnishing
- ❖ Two avocados, halved and thinly sliced

INSTRUCTIONS

1. Preheat the oven to 350°F. Lightly grease a baking sheet with nonstick spray.
2. In a large bowl, toss the zucchini noodles and olive oil to combine—season with salt and Pepper. Divide into four even portions, transfer to the baking sheet and shape each into a nest.
3. Gently crack an egg into the centre of each nest. Bake until the eggs are set, 9 to 11 minutes. Season with salt and pepper; garnish with red pepper flakes and basil. Serve alongside the avocado slices.

207. Pure Indulgence Peanut

Made for: dinner | **Prep Time:** 25 minutes | **Servings:** 02
Per Serving: Kcal: 189, Protein: 7g, Fat: 16g, Net Carb: 6g

INGREDIENTS

- ❖ 1 cup (112g) almond flour.
- ❖ ½ cup (125g) peanut butter (unsweetened). i
- ❖ ⅓ cup (34g) erythritol.
- ❖ 1 tbsp coconut oil.
- ❖ ¾ tsp baking powder.
- ❖ ½ tsp vanilla extract.

INSTRUCTIONS

1. Preheat oven at 350 degrees.
2. In a large bowl, mix all of the ingredients until a dough is formed.
3. Divide the dough into eight large biscuits.
4. Line a baking tray with greaseproof paper.
5. Bake for 10-12 minutes or until golden brown.

208. Cauliflower Rice

Made for: dinner | **Prep Time:** 20 minutes | **Servings:** 02
Per Serving: Kcal: 489, Protein: 24g, Fat: 43g, Net Carb: 3g

INGREDIENTS

Cauliflower rice:
- ❖ 12 oz cauliflower head (grated).
- ❖ 1 ½ oz butter.
- ❖ ¼ tsp turmeric.

- ❖ ¼ tsp salt.

Steak:
- ❖ 1 large 1 inch thick steak (boneless).
- ❖ Two garlic cloves (crushed).
- ❖ 2 tbsp butter.

INSTRUCTIONS

1. In a large frying pan, melt butter. Add cauliflower, salt, and turmeric.
2. Fry for 8-10 minutes or until the cauliflower has softened.
3. Towel dry the steak and rub on salt.
4. In a dry frying pan, sear the steak for 1 minute on each side.
5. Add in butter and garlic. Flip every 30 seconds for 8 minutes (medium-rare), spoon over garlic butter on every flip.
6. Cut steak into strips.

209. Bulky Beef Pie

Made for: dinner | **Prep Time:** 25 minutes | **Servings:** 04
Per Serving: Kcal: 405, Protein: 31g, Fat: 28g, Net Carb: 5g

INGREDIENTS

- ❖ 32 oz minced beef.
- ❖ Six large eggs (whisked).
- ❖ 6 oz tomato puree.
- ❖ 1 ½ cups (170g) cheddar cheese (grated).
- ❖ 2 tbsp dijon mustard.
- ❖ 2 tsp garlic powder.
- ❖ 2 tsp onion powder.
- ❖ 1 tsp salt.
- ❖ 1 tsp olive oil.
- ❖ ½ tsp cayenne pepper.

INSTRUCTIONS

1. Preheat oven at 350 degrees.
2. In a bowl, mix eggs, garlic powder, onion powder, cayenne pepper, and salt. Mix in dijon mustard and tomato puree.
3. In a large frying pan, fry the beef until cooked through. Discard of juices.

4. Allow the beef to slightly cool and then add to the egg mixture; stir well until thoroughly combined. Stir in 1 cup of cheddar cheese.
5. Lightly grease an ovenproof dish and add the mixture. Smooth down and add the remaining cheese.
6. Bake for 30 minutes.
7. Cover and let the pie sit for 15 minutes.

210. Chicken Salad Stuffed

Made for: dinner | **Prep Time:** 20 minutes | **Servings:** 02
Per Serving: Kcal: 116, Protein: 10g, Fat: 14g, Net Carb: 7g

INGREDIENTS

- ⅔ cup (190g) Greek yoghurt
- Two tablespoons Dijon mustard
- Two tablespoons seasoned rice vinegar
- Kosher salt and freshly ground black Pepper
- ⅓ cup (20g) chopped fresh parsley
- Meat from 1 rotisserie chicken, cubed
- Four stalks celery, sliced
- One bunch scallions, sliced and divided
- 1-pint cherry tomatoes, quartered and divided
- ½ English cucumber, diced
- Three bell peppers halved and seeds removed

INSTRUCTIONS

1. In a medium bowl, whisk together the Greek yoghurt, mustard, and rice vinegar; season with salt and Pepper. Stir in the parsley.
2. Add the chicken, celery, and three-quarters each of the scallions, tomatoes, and cucumbers. Stir well to combine.
3. Divide the chicken salad among the bell pepper boats.
4. Garnish with the remaining scallions, tomatoes, and cucumbers.

211. Funky Fried Fish Cakes

Made for: dinner | **Prep Time:** 15 minutes | **Servings:** 04
Per Serving: Kcal: 195, Protein: 13g, Fat: 15g, Net Carb: 1g

INGREDIENTS

- 6 oz mackerel (smoked).
- 4 oz haddock (smoked).
- 4 oz salmon.
- One large egg.
- One garlic clove (crushed).
- 4 tbsp fresh parsley (finely chopped).
- 3 tbsp parmesan (grated).
- 1 tbsp coconut flour.
- 1 tbsp flaxseed (ground).
- 1 ½ oz butter.
- 1 tbsp coconut oil.
- 1 tsp salt.
- 1 tsp chilli flakes.

INSTRUCTIONS

1. Chop all fish into small chunks and mix.
2. In a separate bowl, mix all ingredients except olive oil, coconut oil, and butter.
3. Using your hands, squeeze the mixture until all is combined.
4. Mould the mixture into round, flat balls.
5. In a large frying pan, heat the olive oil, coconut oil, and butter.
6. Fry the fish cakes for 4-5 minutes on each side.

212. Greek bouyiourdi

Made for: dinner | **Prep Time:** 35 minutes | **Servings:** 02
Per Serving: Kcal: 243, Protein: 8g, Fat: 21g, Net Carb: 3g

INGREDIENTS

- 2 large ripe tomatoes
- 1 garlic clove, crushed
- 150g block feta
- 1 large mild green chilli, or 1 green pepper, sliced
- 1 tsp roughly chopped oregano leaves
- 4 tbsp olive oil
- warmed pitta breads, to serve

INSTRUCTIONS

1. Cut 1 tomato through the middle, then cut two slices from the centre and set aside. Scoop the seeds from the rest of the tomato, then grate the flesh, discarding the skin. Deseed and grate the rest of the tomatoes in

the same way, then mix the grated flesh with the garlic. Season and spoon into a 16cm baking dish.

2. Heat the oven to 200C/180C fan/gas 6. Nestle the feta block in the garlicky tomatoes, then top with the sliced tomatoes, the chilli, oregano, olive oil and a pinch of sea salt. Cover the dish and bake for 15 mins, then uncover and bake for a further 15 mins. Serve warm with the pitta breads on the side for dunking.

213. Chicken and Snap

Made for: dinner | **Prep Time:** 15 minutes | **Servings:** 02
Per Serving: Kcal: 228, Protein: 20g, Fat: 11g, Net Carb: 5g

INGREDIENTS

- ❖ Two tablespoons vegetable oil
- ❖ One bunch scallions, thinly sliced
- ❖ Two garlic cloves, minced
- ❖ One red bell pepper, thinly sliced
- ❖ 2½ cups (245 g) snap peas
- ❖ 1¼ cups boneless skinless chicken breast, thinly sliced
- ❖ Salt and freshly ground Black Pepper
- ❖ Three tablespoons soy sauce
- ❖ Two tablespoons rice vinegar
- ❖ Two teaspoons Sriracha (optional)
- ❖ Two tablespoons sesame seeds, plus more for finishing
- ❖ Three tablespoons chopped fresh cilantro, plus more for finishing

INSTRUCTIONS

1. In a large sauté pan, heat the oil over medium heat. Add the scallions and garlic, and sauté until fragrant, about 1 minute. Add the bell pepper and snap peas and sauté until just tender, 2 to 3 minutes.
2. Add the chicken and cook until it is golden and fully cooked, and the vegetables are tender 4 to 5 minutes.
3. Add the soy sauce, rice vinegar, Sriracha (if using), and sesame seeds; toss well to combine. Allow the mixture to simmer for 1 to 2 minutes.

4. Stir in the cilantro, then garnish with a sprinkle of extra cilantro and sesame seeds. Serve immediately.

214. Low Carb Cauliflower

Made for: dinner | **Prep Time:** 25 minutes | **Servings:** 02
Per Serving: Kcal: 185, Protein: 18g, Fat: 18g, Net Carb: 5g

INGREDIENTS

- ❖ Oneihead cauliflower raw
- ❖ 1/2 cup (56g) Mozzarella Cheese shredded
- ❖ 1/2 cup (45g) Parmesan cheese shaved
- ❖ One large egg
- ❖ 1/2 tablespoon garlic minced
- ❖ 1/2 tablespoon fresh basil chopped
- ❖ 1/2 tablespoon fresh Italian flat-leaf parsley chopped
- ❖ One teaspoon salt
- ❖ 1/2 teaspoon ground black pepper
- ❖ 3/4 cup (85g) Mozzarella Cheese shredded

INSTRUCTIONS

1. Preheat oven to 425°F and line a baking sheet with parchment paper or a silicone baking mat.
2. Rice the cauliflower by coring it and breaking it into florets. Then place it in the bowl of a food processor and pulse until it is the texture of rice. (If your cauliflower seems excessively moist, squeeze the riced, raw cauliflower in a paper towel to help remove moisture.)
3. In a large bowl, mix the riced cauliflower, 1/2 cup shredded Mozzarella cheese, 1/2 cup Parmesan cheese, one egg, 1/2 tablespoon fresh garlic, 1/2 tablespoon fresh basil, 1/2 tablespoon fresh parsley, one teaspoon salt, and 1/2 teaspoon black pepper until combined and holds together. Place the mixture onto the lined baking sheet and spread out into a rectangle about 9x7" and 1/4" thick.
4. Bake in the preheated oven for 10-12 minutes. Remove from oven and top with 3/4 cup shredded Mozzarella cheese and return to oven to continue baking until the cheese is melted and starting to brown. Cool

about 10 minutes and cut into 'breadsticks.' Garnish with fresh herbs and Parmesan cheese. Serve with your favourite Red Sauce and enjoy!

215. Garlic Chicken

Made for: dinner | **Prep Time:** 15 minutes | **Servings:** 04
Per Serving: Kcal: 694, Protein: 48g, Fat: 50g, Net Carb: 9g

INGREDIENTS

Cauliflower mash:
- ❖ One large cauliflower head (chopped).
- ❖ One cup (96g) of chicken stock.
- ❖ 3 tbsp butter (cubed).
- ❖ 1 tsp salt.
- ❖ 1 tsp fresh thyme (chopped).

Garlic chicken:
- ❖ 32 oz chicken drumsticks.
- ❖ Six garlic cloves (finely chopped).
- ❖ ½ cup/62g fresh parsley (chopped).
- ❖ 2 oz butter.
- ❖ Juice of 1 lemon.
- ❖ 2 tbsp olive oil.

INSTRUCTIONS

1. Preheat oven at 450 degrees.
2. Place the chicken in a greased ovenproof dish.
3. Drizzle olive oil and lemon juice on the chicken and top with garlic and parsley.
4. Bake for 40-45 minutes or until chicken is thoroughly cooked through and browned. Cauliflower mash:
5. In a large pan, bring chicken stock and salt to boil.
6. Add cauliflower, bring back to boil, reduce heat and simmer for 15-20 minutes, or until cauliflower is tender.
7. Take cauliflower from the pan and add to a blender with 3 tbsp of the stock.
8. Add the butter and thyme; blend until smooth and well combined.

216. Spicy Infused Shrimp

Made for: dinner | **Prep Time:** 15 minutes | **Servings:** 02
Per Serving: Kcal: 257, Protein: 24g, Fat: 17g, Net Carb: 3g

INGREDIENTS

- ❖ 32 oz jumbo shrimp (peeled and deveined).
- ❖ Four garlic cloves (chopped).
- ❖ 1 cup/20g basil leaves.
- ❖ ¼ cup/25g parmesan (grated).
- ❖ ¼ cup/30g walnuts i(chopped).
- ❖ 6 tbsp olive oil.
- ❖ ½ tsp salt.
- ❖ ¼ tsp chilli flakes.

INSTRUCTIONS

1. In a blender, add olive oil, basil, garlic, chilli, salt, parmesan, and walnuts. Blend until well combined.
2. Set 2 tbsp of pesto aside.
3. Add shrimp to the large bowl of pesto and ensure all shrimp are covered. Let marinate for 30-40 minutes.
4. Using cooking spray, spray a wire rack, so it is thoroughly coated.
5. Place shrimp on wire rack and grill for 5 minutes on each side or until slightly charred.
6. Serve the shrimp, using the remaining pesto to taste.

217. Turkey Meatball

Made for: dinner | **Prep Time:** 20 minutes | **Servings:** 04
Per Serving: Kcal: 357, Protein: 24g, Fat: 14g, Net Carb: 6g

INGREDIENTS

- ❖ 1-pound ground turkey
- ❖ One egg, whipped
- ❖ 2-4 tbsp flour (cassava, almond, coconut)
- ❖ Two cloves garlic, crushed (or 1/4 tsp garlic powder) (like this)
- ❖ 2 tbsp fresh herbs (parsley, basil, dill, or cilantro) OR 1/2 tsp dried
- ❖ 3/4 tsp salt
- ❖ several grinds of fresh Black Pepper
- ❖ 2 tbsp butter, ghee, or coconut oil

INSTRUCTIONS

1. In a large bowl, combine turkey meat, egg, flour, garlic, salt, and herbs and mix until well incorporated. Roll into small balls (about 1 1/2 inches). You'll get about 24-26 meatballs—heat 2 tbsp fat of choice in a large skillet on medium-high heat.
2. Cook meatballs for 3-4 minutes, until all sides are brown. You may need to do this in batches. Set aside.

218. Mighty Meaty Moussaka

Made for: dinner | **Prep Time:** 25 minutes | **Servings:** 04
Per Serving: Kcal: 742, Protein: 43g, Fat: 59g, Net Carb: 4g

INGREDIENTS

- ❖ 20 oz minced beef.
- ❖ One medium aubergine (thinly sliced).
- ❖ One onion (finely chopped).
- ❖ Two garlic cloves (crushed).
- ❖ ½ cup/110g tomato puree.
- ❖ 4 tbsp olive oil.
- ❖ 1 tbsp paprika powder.
- ❖ 1 tsp salt.
- ❖ ½ tsp black pepper.
- ❖ ½ tsp cinnamon (ground).

Cheese sauce:
- ❖ 7 oz swiss cheese (grated).
- ❖ 3 oz cream cheese.
- ❖ ½ cup/115g of thick cream/double cram.
- ❖ One garlic clove (crushed).
- ❖ ¼ tsp salt.

INSTRUCTIONS

1. Preheat oven at 350 degrees.
2. In a large frying pan, fry the auberge slices until golden brown and softened. Set to one side.
3. In the same pan, cook the minced beef until browned. Add onion, garlic, and spices; pour in the tomato puree and simmer for 5 minutes.

4. In a pan, mix the cheese sauce ingredients (only using half of the swiss cheese). Stirring continuously, Simmer until sauce thickens.
5. Pour meat sauce into an ovenproof dish, layer the auberges on top and pour on the cheese sauce. Sprinkle the remaining swiss cheese on top.
6. Bake for 20-25 minutes or until cheese turns golden brown.

219. Creamy Keto Chicken

Made for: dinner | **Prep Time:** 15 minutes | **Servings:** 04
Per Serving: Kcal: 758, Protein: 40g, Fat: 64g, Net Carb: 7g

INGREDIENTS

- ❖ 32 oz chicken thighs (boneless and skinless).
- ❖ 16 oz cauliflower (florets).
- ❖ 7 oz cheddar cheese (grated).
- ❖ 4 oz cherry tomatoes (halved).
- ❖ 1 ½ oz butter.
- ❖ One leek (chopped).
- ❖ ¾ cup (180g) sour cream.
- ❖ ½ cup (55g) of cream cheese (softened).
- ❖ 3 tbsp pesto.
- ❖ 3 tbsp lemon juice (fresh).
- ❖ ½ tsp black pepper.

INSTRUCTIONS

1. Preheat oven at 400 degrees.
2. In a large frying pan, melt the butter and fry chicken until cooked and golden brown.
3. In ia bowl, mix sour cream, cream cheese, lemon juice, pesto, and Pepper until well icombined.
4. Place chicken in a large ovenproof dish, pour cream cheese mixture on top.
5. Add cauliflower, leek, and tomatoes.
6. Bake in the oven for 25 minutes, remove and sprinkle cheese on top.
7. Bake for a further 10 minutes or until cheese is melted and golden brown.

220. Chicken Chasseur

Made for: dinner | **Prep Time:** 15 minutes | **Servings:** 04
Per Serving: Kcal: 570, Protein: 31g, Fat: 48g, Net Carb: 3g

INGREDIENTS

- ❖ 16 oz chicken breast.
- ❖ 8 oz baby mushrooms.
- ❖ Four cloves garlic (crushed).
- ❖ ½ red onion (finely chopped).
- ❖ 1 ½ cups (350g) thick cream/double cream
- ❖ ¼ cup (22g) parmesan (grated).
- ❖ 2 tbsp butter (unsalted).
- ❖ 1 tbsp olive oil.
- ❖ 1 tsp mixed herbs (dried).
- ❖ 1 tsp garlic powder.
- ❖ ¼ tsp salt.
- ❖ ¼ tsp black pepper.

INSTRUCTIONS

1. Slice chicken breasts in half (lengthways), making them easier to cook.
2. In a bowl, mix garlic powder, mixed herbs, salt, and Pepper. Season both sides of chicken breasts with the mixture.
3. In a large frying pan, melt the butter. Fry the chicken breasts, 5 minutes on each side or until thoroughly cooked. Set cooked chicken to one side.
4. Using the same frying pan, add mushrooms and onion; fry until tender and slightly browned. Add crushed garlic and cook for an additional minute.
5. Reduce heat and stir in the thick cream, parmesan, and herbs; simmer until sauce begins to thicken, stirring continuously.
6. Return chicken and any juices back to the pan, cook for an additional 3-4 minutes.

221. Spicy Salmon with Salsa

Made for: dinner | **Prep Time:** 15 minutes | **Servings:** 02
Per Serving: Kcal: 444, Protein: 35g, Fat: 32g, Net Carb: 6g

INGREDIENTS

- ❖ 4 salmon fillets.
- ❖ 1 tbsp olive oil.
- ❖ 4 tsp cajun seasoning.
- ❖ Two avocados (chopped into small chunks).
- ❖ One jalapeno (finely chopped).
- ❖ One red onion (finely chopped).
- ❖ 1 tbsp lime juice (fresh).
- ❖ 1 tbsp fresh coriander (finely chopped).

INSTRUCTIONS

1. Season both sides of salmon with Cajun seasoning.
2. Heat the oil in a large frying pan and fry the salmon until extremely golden brown; turn and repeat for the other side.
3. Mix the avocados, jalapenos, onion, coriander, and lime until well combined.
4. Serve with salmon.

222. Cashew Chicken

Made for: dinner | **Prep Time:** 15 minutes | **Servings:** 02
Per Serving: Kcal: 655, Protein: 17g, Fat: 56g, Net Carb: 8g

INGREDIENTS

- ❖ Three raw chicken thighs boneless, skinless
- ❖ 2 tbsp coconut oil (for cooking)
- ❖ 1/4 cup (35g) raw cashews
- ❖ 1/2 medium Green Bell Pepper
- ❖ 1/2 tsp ground ginger
- ❖ 1 tbsp rice wine vinegar
- ❖ 1 1/2 tbsp liquid aminos
- ❖ 1/2 tbsp chilli garlic sauce
- ❖ 1 tbsp minced garlic
- ❖ 1 tbsp Sesame Oil
- ❖ 1 tbsp Sesame Seeds
- ❖ 1 tbsp green onions
- ❖ 1/4 medium white onion
- ❖ Salt + Pepper

INSTRUCTIONS

1. Heat a pan over low heat and toast the cashews for 8 minutes or until they start to lightly brown and become fragrant. Remove and set aside.
2. Dice chicken thighs into 1-inch chunks. Cut onion and Pepper into equally large pieces.
3. Increase heat to high and add coconut oil to the pan.
4. Once the oil is up to temperature, add in the chicken thighs and allow them to cook through (about 5 minutes).

5. Once the chicken is fully cooked, add in the Pepper, onions, garlic, chilli garlic sauce, and seasonings (ginger, salt, Pepper). Allow cooking on high for 2-3 minutes.
6. Add liquid amino, rice wine vinegar, and cashews. Cook on high and allow the liquid to reduce down until it is a sticky consistency, there should not be excess liquid in the pan upon completing cooking.
7. Serve in a bowl, top with sesame seeds and drizzle with sesame oil. Enjoy!

223. Garlic Chicken Kebab

Made for: dinner | **Prep Time:** 15 minutes | **Servings:** 04
Per Serving: Kcal: 276, Protein: 33g, Fat: 14g, Net Carb: 2g

INGREDIENTS

- ❖ 32 oz chicken breast (cut into 1 inch cubes).
- ❖ Four garlic cloves (crushed).
- ❖ One lemon (zested and juiced).
- ❖ ½ cup (55g) of almond milk.
- ❖ ¼ cup (60ml) olive oil.
- ❖ ¼ cup (15g) fresh parsley (finely ichopped).
- ❖ ½ tsp salt.
- ❖ ¼ tsp black pepper.
- ❖ 1 tbsp mixed herbs (dried).

INSTRUCTIONS

1. In a large bowl, mix garlic, lemon, almond milk, olive oil, parsley, salt, Pepper, and herbs.
2. Add chicken cubes to the bowl and stir well to ensure all chicken is coated.
3. Chill in the fridge for 2-3 hours, occasionally stirring to ensure even coverage.
4. Fry the chicken in a large frying pan until browned and cooked through.
5. Using wooden skewers, fill the skewer with chicken pieces.

224. Antipasto Meat Sticks

Made for: dinner | **Prep Time:** 15 minutes | **Servings:** 02
Per Serving: Kcal: 234, Protein: 10g, Fat: 21g, Net Carb: 1g

INGREDIENTS

- ❖ 4 slices salami.
- ❖ Four slices sandwich ham.
- ❖ Four slices pepperoni.
- ❖ 4 slices cheddar cheese.
- ❖ Four slices mozzarella.
- ❖ One handful lettuce (chopped)
- ❖ 2 tbsp olive oil.
- ❖ 1 tbsp apple cider vinegar.
- ❖ 1 tbsp mayonnaise.
- ❖ ½ tsp mixed herbs (dried).

INSTRUCTIONS

1. In 4 separate piles, layer the meat slices from biggest to smallest.
2. Spread with mayonnaise and add the cheese slices.
3. Sprinkle on lettuce.
4. Roll each pile into a tight sausage shape; secure with a toothpick.
5. In a dish, add olive oil, vinegar, and herbs to use as a dip for antipasto sticks.

225. Spicy Tuna Sushi Rolls

Made for: dinner | **Prep Time:** 15 minutes | **Servings:** 02
Per Serving: Kcal: 123, Protein: 10g, Fat: 9g, Net Carb: 2g

INGREDIENTS

- ❖ 1 cucumber.
- ❖ ½ can tuna (in olive oil).
- ❖ ½ avocado (sliced).
- ❖ 1 tsp chilli sauce.
- ❖ ¼ tsp salt.
- ❖ ¼ tsp black pepper.
- ❖ Pinch of cayenne Pepper.

INSTRUCTIONS

1. Using a potato peeler, thinly slice cucumber (lengthways) until the outer layer has gone. Discard the outer layer and thinly slice the cucumber until you have six long strips.
2. In a medium bowl, mix tuna, chilli sauce, Salt, Pepper, and cayenne until well combined.
3. Take a cucumber slice and spoon the mixture over, leaving half an inch at each end.

4. Place 1-2 pieces of avocado on each cucumber slice and carefully roll.
5. Use a toothpick to secure.

226. Loaded Cauliflower

Made for: dinner | **Prep Time:** 20 minutes | **Servings:** 02
Per Serving: Kcal: 298, Protein: 11g, Fat: 24g, Net Carb: 7g

INGREDIENTS

- ❖ 1 pound cauliflower
- ❖ 4 ounces sour cream
- ❖ 1 cup/110g grated cheddar cheese
- ❖ Two slices bacon cooked and crumbled
- ❖ Two tablespoons chives snipped
- ❖ Three tablespoons butter
- ❖ 1/4 teaspoon garlic powder
- ❖ salt and Pepper to taste

INSTRUCTIONS

1. Cut the cauliflower into florets and add them to a microwave-safe bowl. Add two tablespoons of water and cover with cling film. Microwave for 5-8 minutes, depending on your microwave, until thoroughly cooked and tender. Drain the excess water and let sit uncovered for a minute or two. (Alternately, steam your cauliflower the conventional way. You may need to squeeze a little water out of the cauliflower after cooking.)
2. Add the cauliflower to a food processor and process until fluffy. Add the butter, garlic powder, and sour cream and process until it resembles the consistency of mashed potatoes. Remove the mashed cauliflower to a bowl and add most of the chives, saving some to add to the top later. Add half of the cheddar cheese and mix by hand—season with salt and Pepper.
3. Top the loaded cauliflower with the remaining cheese, remaining chives, and bacon. Put back into the microwave to melt the cheese or place the cauliflower under the broiler for a few minutes.

227. Creamy Cauliflower

Made for: dinner | **Prep Time:** 20 minutes | **Servings:** 02
Per Serving: Kcal: 216, Protein: 5g, Fat: 14g, Net Carb: 6g

INGREDIENTS

- ❖ One tablespoon butter
- ❖ 1/2 cup (70g) diced Onion
- ❖ 5 Garlic Cloves (minced)
- ❖ 1/2 cup (64g) diced Carrots
- ❖ 1 Whole Head of Cauliflower (cut into small florets)
- ❖ 1 1/2 cups (370g) Vegetable Broth
- ❖ One teaspoon freshly ground Pepper
- ❖ 1/2 teaspoon dried Oregano
- ❖ 1/4 cup (55g) cream cheese
- ❖ Salt to taste
- ❖ Olive Oil and cooked bacon for topping

INSTRUCTIONS

1. In a dutch oven or soup pot, heat butter and add onions and garlic.
2. Saute for a few minutes till the onions are soft.
3. Add carrots, cauliflower, vegetable broth, pepper, oregano, and salt to the pot. Bring this to a boil, and slow the heat down to a simmer. Cook for 15 minutes or so till the cauliflower is tender.
4. Switch off the flame and using a blender, blend the soup partly in the soup pot. If you don't have a hand blender, pour half the soup into a blender and pulse a few tips till creamy.
5. Switch the flame back on and add a cup of water or broth along with the cream cheese. Simmer for 5-10 minutes and switch off the flame. Feel free to thin the soup further if you like with some more broth or milk. Top with olive oil and bacon and serve hot.

228. Tasty Salted Turnip Fries

Made for: dinner | **Prep Time:** 15 minutes | **Servings:** 02
Per Serving: Kcal: 219, Protein: 2g, Fat: 22g, Net Carb: 7g

INGREDIENTS

- ❖ 16 oz turnips.

- ❖ 6 tbsp olive oil.
- ❖ 2 tsp onion powder.
- ❖ ½ tsp paprika.
- ❖ 1 tsp salt.

INSTRUCTIONS

1. Preheat oven at 400 degrees.
2. Wash and peel the turnips; cut into ½ inch strips.
3. In a large bowl, toss the turnips in 2 tbsp of olive oil, salt, onion powder, and paprika.
4. Add remaining oil to a baking tray and heat in the oven for 5 minutes.
5. Bake for 25-30 minutes or until fries are golden brown and crispy.

229. Tantalizingly Tasty

Made for: dinner | **Prep Time:** 15 minutes | **Servings:** 04
Per Serving: Kcal: 180, Protein: 12g, Fat: 18g, Net Carb: 3g

INGREDIENTS

- ❖ 8 oz cream cheese (softened).
- ❖ Two cans' tomatoes (chopped).
- ❖ Four cups (390 g) of chicken broth.
- ❖ One cup (90 g) parmesan (grated).
- ❖ ½ cup (75 g) red onions (finely chopped).
- ❖ 2 tbsp coconut oil.
- ❖ Two garlic cloves (crushed).
- ❖ 1 tbsp basil (dried).
- ❖ 1 tsp oregano (dried).
- ❖ 1 tsp salt.
- ❖ ½ tsp black pepper.

INSTRUCTIONS

1. In a large pan, place the coconut oil, onions, garlic, basil, and oregano; cook over medium heat until onions are softened.
2. Add in cream cheese, stirring continuously.
3. Gradually add the broth, tomatoes, parmesan, salt, and Pepper.
4. Cover and simmer for 8-10 minutes.
5. Pour soup into a blender and blend until pureed.

230. Eggs with Asparagus

Made for: dinner | Prep
Per Serving: Kcal: 288, P.

INGREDIENTS

- ❖ 2 pounds asparagus
- ❖ 1-pint cherry tomatoes
- ❖ Four eggs
- ❖ Two tablespoons olive oil
- ❖ Two teaspoons chopped fresh thyme
- ❖ Salt and Pepper to taste

INSTRUCTIONS

1. Preheat the oven to 400°F. Grease a baking sheet with non-stick cooking spray.
2. Arrange the asparagus and cherry tomatoes in an even layer on the baking sheet. Drizzle the olive oil over the vegetables; season with the thyme and salt and Pepper to taste.
3. Roast in the oven until the asparagus is nearly tender and the tomatoes are wrinkled, 10 to 12 minutes.
4. Crack the eggs on top of the asparagus; season each with salt and Pepper.
5. Return to the oven and bake until the egg whites are set but the yolks are still jiggly, 7 to 8 minutes more.
6. To serve, divide the asparagus, tomatoes, and eggs among four plates.

231. Greek Wedge Salad

Made for: dinner | **Prep Time:** 15 minutes | **Servings:** 04
Per Serving: Kcal: 248, Protein: 0g, Fat: 27g, Net Carb: 1g

INGREDIENTS

- ❖ ½ cup (120 ml) extra-virgin olive oil
- ❖ One tablespoon Dijon mustard
- ❖ One garlic clove, minced
- ❖ One teaspoon dried oregano
- ❖ One teaspoon salt
- ❖ ¾ teaspoon freshly ground Black Pepper
- ❖ ⅓ cup (80 ml) red wine vinegar

INSTRUCTIONS

1. In a medium bowl, whisk the olive oil with

232. Perfect almond Cake

Made for: dinner | **Prep Time:** 50 minutes | **Servings:** 02
Per Serving: Kcal: 300, Protein: 10g, Fat: 28g, Net Carb: 6g

INGREDIENTS

- ❖ 4 large eggs.
- ❖ 1 ½ cups (170g) almond flour.
- ❖ ¾ cup (170g) pumpkin puree (canned).
- ❖ ⅔ cup (65g) erythritol.
- ❖ ½ cup (125g) softened butter.
- ❖ ½ cup (55g) coconut flour.
- ❖ 4 tsp baking powder.
- ❖ 1 tsp vanilla extract.
- ❖ 1 tsp cinnamon (ground).
- ❖ ½ tsp nutmeg (ground).
- ❖ ½ tsp salt.
- ❖ ¼ tsp ginger (ground).

INSTRUCTIONS

1. Preheat oven at 350 degrees.
2. Mix the butter and erythritol until light and creamy.
3. One at a time, whisk in eggs until all ingredients are well combined.
4. Mix in pumpkin puree and vanilla.
5. In another bowl, mix the almond flour, baking powder, coconut flour, cinnamon, nutmeg, ginger, and salt.
6. Add the flour mixture to the egg mixture; stir until well combined.
7. Line a 9 x 5-inch loaf pan with greaseproof paper and pour in the butter mixture.
8. Bake for 45 -50 minutes or until a skewer inserted in the middle comes out clean.

233. Overnight Oats

Made for: dinner | **Prep Time:** 15 minutes | **Servings:** 02

INSTRUCTIONS

1. Place rolled oats, chia seeds, and flax seeds in a large bowl. Poor in 2 ½ cups of strawberry cashew milk (or preferred dairy, nut or seed milk) and stir well to combine. Cover and store in the fridge for 1 hour or overnight.
2. Check consistency and add additional Strawberry Cashew Milk as desired. Portion into individual containers. Add fresh strawberries, cashews, chia seeds, flax seeds, or extra Strawberry Cashew Milk as toppings. Enjoy immediately or store in airtight containers for up to 5 days.

234. Strawberry Cashew Milk

Made for: dinner | **Prep Time:** 20 minutes | **Servings:** 04
Per Serving: Kcal: 516, Protein: 27g, Fat: 44g, Net Carb: 5g

INGREDIENTS

- ❖ 2 cups (280g) raw, unsalted cashews
- ❖ 1 pint of strawberries (2-2 ½ cups)
- ❖ 4 cups (900ml) of filtered water
- ❖ Pinch of sea salt

INSTRUCTIONS

1. Using a high-speed blender, add cashews and water to the pitcher.
2. While cashews are soaking, wash strawberries, trim to tops, and slice in half.
3. Add strawberries, sea salt, and optional sweetener. Blend on high for 1 minute till full incorporated and smooth.
4. Store in an airtight container in the fridge for up to 7 days.

235. Continental pie

Made for: dinner | **Prep Time:** 25 minutes | **Servings:** 02
Per Serving: Kcal: 1069, Protein: 81g, Fat: 96g, Net Carb: 4g

INGREDIENTS

Bread roll:
- ❖ 3 large eggs.
- ❖ 1 ½ cups (170g) mozzarella (grated).
- ❖ One ⅓ cups (150g) almond flour.
- ❖ 2 oz cream cheese (full fat).
- ❖ 2 tbsp coconut flour.
- ❖ 1 ½ tbsp baking powder.

Continental:
- ❖ One egg (hard-boiled).
- ❖ One slice ham (smoked).
- ❖ One cup cheddar cheese (grated).
- ❖ Two slices salami.
- ❖ Three slices mozzarella.

INSTRUCTIONS

1. Preheat oven at 350 degrees.
2. Mix almond flour, coconut flour, and baking powder. Set aside.
3. In a separate bowl (microwave-safe), add mozzarella and cream cheese, cover, and melt for 30 seconds. Stir. Repeat for an additional 30 seconds, and a dough has formed.
4. Allow dough to cool slightly (so it's still warm to the touch but not hot).
5. Add dough, two eggs, and flour mixture to a blender; blend on high speed until a sticky dough has formed.
6. Place the sticky dough onto a piece of cling film and cover. Knead the dough (while in cling film) until it is completely uniform.
7. Divide the dough into eight equal pieces and roll them into smooth balls.
8. Line a baking tray with greaseproof paper and place the balls 2 inches apart.
9. Take the final egg and whisk in a bowl; brush the rolls with the glaze.
10. Bake for 20-22 minutes or until golden brown.
11. On a serving plate, add the slices of salami, a slice of smoked ham, mozzarella, hard-boiled egg, and cheddar cheese. Place the hot bread roll on the side.

236. Spicy Kick-Start

Made for: dinner | **Prep Time:** 20 minutes | **Servings:** 02
Per Serving: Kcal: 689, Protein: 35g, Fat: 60g, Net Carb: 4g

INGREDIENTS

- ❖ 4 large eggs.
- ❖ 8 oz can of mackerel in tomato sauce.
- ❖ ½ red onion (finely sliced).
- ❖ ¼ cup (60ml) olive oil.
- ❖ 2 oz lettuce.
- ❖ 2 tbsp butter.
- ❖ Salt and pepper.

INSTRUCTIONS

1. Melt butter in a frying pan and cook the eggs to your preference.
2. On a serving plate, place lettuce and top with onion. Add the eggs and mackerel to the plate.
3. Drizzle olive oil over the lettuce and season with salt and pepper.

237. Keto-Classic Cereal

Made for: dinner | **Prep Time:** 25 minutes | **Servings:** 04
Per Serving: Kcal: 207, Protein: 6g, Fat: 18g, Net Carb: 3g

INGREDIENTS

- ❖ 1 cup (110g) almond flour.
- ❖ 2 tbsp water.
- ❖ 2 tbsp sunflower seeds.
- ❖ 1 tbsp coconut oil.
- ❖ 1 tbsp flaxseed meal.
- ❖ 1 tsp vanilla extract.
- ❖ 1 tsp cinnamon (ground).
- ❖ ¼ tsp salt.

INSTRUCTIONS

1. Preheat oven at 350 degrees.

2. Add almond flour, sunflower seeds, flaxseed meal, cinnamon, and salt to a blender and blend until sunflower seeds are finely chopped.
3. Mix in the water and coconut oil and blend until a dough is formed.
4. Place dough on a piece of greaseproof paper and press flat. Place another piece of greaseproof paper on top and roll the dough until it is approximately 3mm in thickness.
5. Remove top paper and cut the dough into 1-inch squares.
6. Place the greaseproof paper (with the cut squares) on to a baking tray.
7. Bake in the oven for 10-15 minutes or until lightly browned and crisp.
8. Allow to cool and then separate the squares.
9. Serve with unsweetened almond milk.

238. Mushroom baked

Made for: dinner | **Prep Time:** 15 minutes | **Servings:** 02
Per Serving: Kcal: 578, Protein: 30g, Fat: 47g, Net Carb: 4g

INGREDIENTS:

- ❖ 2 large deep cup mushrooms (stem removed).
- ❖ Four slices of bacon (cooked and chopped).
- ❖ Two large eggs.
- ❖ 1/10 cup (9g) parmesan (grated).
- ❖ Cooking spray.

INSTRUCTIONS

1. Preheat oven at 375 degrees.
2. On a baking tray, spray the mushrooms with cooking spray and bake for 10 minutes.
3. Split the bacon and parmesan between the two mushrooms and bake for an additional 5 minutes.
4. Crack an egg into each mushroom and bake for an additional 10 minutes.

239. Keto Pancakes

Made for: dinner | **Prep Time:** 15 minutes | **Servings:** 04
Per Serving: Kcal: 111, Protein: 5g, Fat: 12g, Net Carb: 2g

INGREDIENTS

- ❖ 1/2 cup (112g) almond flour
- ❖ 4 oz. cream cheese, softened
- ❖ 4 large eggs
- ❖ 1 tsp. lemon zest
- ❖ Butter, for frying and serving

INSTRUCTIONS

1. In a medium bowl, whisk together almond flour, cream cheese, eggs, and lemon zest until smooth.
2. In a nonstick skillet over medium-low heat, melt 1 tablespoon butter. Pour in about 3 tablespoons batter and cook until golden, 2 minutes. Flip and cook 2 minutes more. Transfer to a plate and repeat with remaining batter.
3. Serve topped with butter.

240. Baked Egg

Made for: dinner | **Prep Time:** 20 minutes | **Servings:** 02
Per Serving: Kcal: 498, Protein: 40g, Fat: 36g, Net Carb: 2g

INGREDIENTS:

- ❖ 2 large eggs.
- ❖ 3 oz minced beef.
- ❖ 2 oz cheddar cheese (grated).

INSTRUCTIONS

1. Preheat oven at 400 degrees.
2. Put the minced beef into a baking dish; make two holes in the mince and crack in the eggs.
3. Sprinkle the cheese over the top.
4. Bake for 10-15 minutes or until the eggs are cooked.

241. Cobb Salad

Made for: dinner | **Prep Time:** 15 minutes | **Servings:** 02
Per Serving: Kcal: 602, Protein: 41g, Fat: 40g, Net Carb: 2g

INGREDIENTS

- ❖ 1 cup (30g) spinach
- ❖ 1 hard boiled egg

- ❖ 2 strips bacon
- ❖ 2 oz. chicken breast
- ❖ 1/2 campari tomato
- ❖ 1/4 avocado
- ❖ 1/2 tsp white vinegar
- ❖ 1 tbsp olive oil

INSTRUCTIONS

1. Cook your bacon and chicken if they are not yet cooked. Shred your chicken or slice it any way you prefer.
2. Chop up all your ingredients into bite sized pieces.
3. Combine them in a large mixing bowl with your oil and vinegar (you can also use a low carb bleu cheese dressing!).
4. Toss well and enjoy!

242. Shredded Fennel Salad

Made for: dinner | **Prep Time:** 25 minutes | **Servings:** 04
Per Serving: Kcal: 436, Protein: 77g, Fat: 61g, Net Carb: 3g

INGREDIENTS

- ❖ 4 cups (900g) mixed salad greens or 5 oz container
- ❖ One fennel, fronds removed (1 cup shredded)
- ❖ ¼ red cabbage, shredded (1 cup shredded)
- ❖ 1/8 red onion (1/4 cup)
- ❖ ½ cup fresh herbs, such as mint, parsley, and cilantro
- ❖ Two chicken breasts
- ❖ 1 Tbsp Adobo Spice Mix
- ❖ Whipped Lemon Vinaigrette

INSTRUCTIONS

1. Preheat grill on high. Season chicken evenly with a spice mix. Grill on medium-high for 10 minutes, turning halfway through. Set aside to cool.
2. Prepare the salad by rough chopping mixed greens and place equally in two salad bowls. Using a mandolin, shave fennel bulb on the first or mini-setting of your mandolin, along with the red onion. If slicing with a knife, slice ¼ inch thin or thinner. Slice fennel shreds in half and toss with greens.

3. Shave the red cabbage on the other mandolin setting for ¼ inch slices. Mix with greens and fennel. Add fresh mint, parsley, dill, or cilantro. Lightly toss with Whipped Lemon Vinaigrette. Finish with sliced chicken breast. Garnish with avocado, feta, or goat cheese if desired. Holds well for meal prep for five days.

243. Keto Coconut Macaroons

Prep Time: 15 minutes | **Servings:** 20 Cookies
Per Cookies: Kcal: 31, Protein: 0.8g, Fat: 2g, Net Carb: 1g

INGREDIENTS

- ❖ 3 egg whites' medium-sized, at room temperature
- ❖ 2 cups (180g) of shredded coconut
- ❖ 1/3 cup (8 g) Sweetener

INSTRUCTIONS

1. Preheat oven to 320°F (160°C). Line a big baking sheet with parchment paper.
2. Separate egg whites from egg yolks and put all the whites into a large bowl.
3. Whip the egg whites with a hand mixer until they have stiff peaks. This should take around 3-5 minutes.
4. Carefully fold in the shredded coconut and sweetener to the egg whites being careful not to over mix too much.
5. Take a 1 tablespoon measuring spoon and with that, scoop out small portions of the cookies, shaping them into balls as you go. Place them on your baking tray with about 1/2 inch in between each macaroon, they won't rise much so don't worry about leaving big gaps. This recipe should make about 20 cookies.
6. Bake for 17-20 minutes until they are golden and crispy.

244. Chicken Bacon Ranch

Made for: dinner | **Prep Time:** 10 minutes | **Servings:** 02
Per Serving: Kcal: 329, Protein: 19g, Fat: 21g, Net Carb: 3g

INGREDIENTS

- ❖ 6 slices of mozzarella cheese
- ❖ 1 1/2 cups (210g) cooked shredded or grilled chicken
- ❖ 1/4 cup (55g) cooked bacon (2-3 slices cooked)
- ❖ 1 tablespoon low carb ranch dressing
- ❖ 1 teaspoon green onion, chopped

INSTRUCTIONS

1. Combine the chicken, bacon, ranch and green onions, set aside.
2. Preheat your oven to 350 degrees. Line a large baking sheet with a silicone baking mat.
3. Place the mozzarella slices on the silicone baking sheet. Bake 5-7 minutes.
4. When the edges have browned and the cheese is bubbly (watch the video if you need some guidance) remove from the oven. Allow them to cool about 1 minute, just so they cool enough you can handle, but still very pliable.
5. Place the chicken bacon ranch mixture on the edge of one slice and tightly roll them up, seam side down.

245. Sandwich Lunchbox

Made for: dinner | **Prep Time:** 15 minutes | **Servings:** 04
Per Serving: Kcal: 578, Protein: 29g, Fat: 58g, Net Carb: 6g

INGREDIENTS

- ❖ 2 Slices Genoa Salami
- ❖ 12 Slices Ham
- ❖ 12 slices Pepperoni
- ❖ 12 Slices Provolone
- ❖ 6 tbsp Mayo
- ❖ 1/2 cup (35g) Shredded Lettuce
- ❖ 40 black olives
- ❖ 2 apples

INSTRUCTIONS

1. Lay ingredients on cutting board and roll sandwich up. Secure with a toothpick.

2. Place your ingredients into your EasyLunchboxes. Cover and refrigerate until ready to use. Use within 3 days.

246. Keto-Buzz Blueberry

Made for: dinner | **Prep Time:** 20 minutes | **Servings:** 02
Per Serving: Kcal: 132, Protein: 7g, Fat: 7g, Net Carb: 4g

INGREDIENTS

- ❖ Three large eggs.
- ❖ ½ cup (55g) almond iflour.
- ❖ ¼ cup (60ml) of imilk.
- ❖ ¼ cup (50g) of fresh blueberries.
- ❖ 2 tbsp coconut flour.
- ❖ 2 tbsp sweetener (granulated).
- ❖ 1 tsp cinnamon (ground).
- ❖ ½ tsp baking powder.

INSTRUCTIONS

1. Add all ingredients (except blueberries) to a blender and mix until a thick batter is formed.
2. Add the blended mixture to a bowl and stir in blueberries.
3. Grease a large non-stick frying pan and allow the pot to get hot over medium heat.
4. Pour ¼ cup of the mixture into the hot pan, allow to cook for 2 - 3 minutes, or until the edges start to crisp and turn lightly browned. Flip and repeat.
5. Repeat the process using the remaining batter.

247. Perfect Mozzarella

Made for: dinner | **Prep Time:** 15 minutes | **Servings:** 02
Per Serving: Kcal: 258, Protein: 16g, Fat: 18g, Net Carb: 7g

INGREDIENTS

- ❖ 3 eggs.
- ❖ 8 oz mozzarella (grated).
- ❖ 4 oz bacon (grilled).
- ❖ 2 oz cream cheese.
- ❖ ⅔ cup (75g) almond flour.
- ❖ ½ cup (56g) cheddar cheese (grated).
- ❖ ⅓ cup (38g) coconut flour.

- ❖ 2 tsp baking powder.
- ❖ 1 tsp salt.

INSTRUCTIONS

1. Preheat oven at 350 degrees.
2. Microwave the cream cheese and mozzarella for 60 seconds. Stir and microwave for an additional 60 seconds.
3. Put one egg, almond flour, coconut flour, baking powder, and salt into a blender and pour in the melted cheese mixture. Blend until a dough forms.
4. Split the dough into eight pieces. Flatten each piece to form a 5-inch circle, place on a baking tray lined with baking paper.
5. Scramble the remaining two eggs and divide between each circle; do the same with bacon and cheddar cheese.
6. Fold the edges in and seal the semi-circle using fingertips.
7. Bake for 20 minutes or until lightly browned.

248. What Waffle!

Made for: dinner | **Prep Time:** 25 minutes | **Servings:** 02
Per Serving: Kcal: 345, Protein: 11g, Fat: 31g, Net Carb: 8g

INGREDIENTS

- ❖ 2 large eggs.
- ❖ 2 cups almond flour.
- ❖ 1 ½ cups (360 ml) almond milk (warm).
- ❖ ⅓ cup (80 g) butter (melted).
- ❖ 2 tbsp erythritol.
- ❖ 4 tsp baking powder.
- ❖ 1 tsp vanilla extract.
- ❖ 1 itsp salt.

INSTRUCTIONS

1. Mix baking powder, salt, and almond flour until well combined.
2. In a separate bowl, whisk the eggs until well combined.
3. Take the lukewarm almond milk and mix with the eggs, adding melted butter, erythritol, and vanilla extract.

4. Stir the egg mixture into the flour mixture until a dough is formed. Let sit for several minutes.
5. Cook in a hot waffle iron for 6-8 minutes.

249. Chile Relleno Casserole

Made for: dinner | **Prep Time:** 40 minutes | **Servings:** 04
Per Serving: Kcal: 421, Protein: 26g, Fat: 33g, Net Carb: 3g

INGREDIENTS

- ❖ ½ lb ground beef, lean
- ❖ ½ cup (75g) onions, diced
- ❖ 8 oz diced or whole roasted chiles or 2 ifresh poblanos, roasted and peeled
- ❖ 1 cup (110g) sharp cheddar cheese, shredded
- ❖ ½ cup (60g) monterey jack cheese, ishredded
- ❖ 2 eggs
- ❖ ½ cup (115g) heavy cream/double cream
- ❖ ¾ teaspoon cumin
- ❖ ¼ teaspoon salt
- ❖ ⅛ teaspoon pepper

INSTRUCTIONS

1. Preheat oven to 375 degrees.
2. Brown ground beef with onion and sprinkle with salt and pepper as desired.
3. In an 8 X 8 oven proof baking dish, layer chiles. Next add layer of ground beef onion mixture. Next add layer of cheddar and monterey jack cheese.
4. Whisk together remaining ingredients then pour over casserole. Bake in preheated oven for 20 minutes or until mixture is set and cheese is golden and bubbly.
5. Serve immediately with salsa and sour cream if desired.

250. Keto Bacon Wrapped

Made for: dinner | **Prep Time:** 20 minutes | **Servings:** 02
Per Serving: Kcal: 386, Protein: 35g, Fat: 81g, Net Carb: 3g

INGREDIENTS

- ❖ 1 lb (450g) extra-large raw shrimp - peeled, deveined, tail on
- ❖ sea salt and pepper - to taste

- ❖ 1/4 tsp chilli powder
- ❖ 1/4 tsp cayenne pepper
- ❖ 1 tsp smoked paprika
- ❖ 1 Tbsp fresh lemon juice
- ❖ 1 Tbsp olive oil
- ❖ 6-8 very thin slices of bacon - (about 12 oz. / 340g)

Keto white Sauce:
- ❖ 1 cup (240g) mayonnaise
- ❖ 1 Tbsp dijon mustard
- ❖ 2 tsp prepared horseradish
- ❖ 2 Tbsp apple cider vinegar
- ❖ 1 tsp garlic powder
- ❖ sea salt and pepper - to taste

INSTRUCTIONS

1. Preheat the oven to 400°F (200°C) and line a large baking tray with parchment paper.
2. Place the raw shrimp into a bowl and sprinkle with seasonings. Drizzle olive oil and fresh lemon juice and gently toss to coat.
3. Cut the bacon strips in half and wrap each shrimp in one bacon half-slice. Insert a toothpick through the bacon to secure the wrap.
4. Arrange the shrimp in a single layer on the prepared pan. Roast the bacon-wrapped shrimp for 10-12 minutes, flipping it halfway.
5. Meanwhile, combine all sauce ingredients in a jug and whisk to emulsify. Refrigerate until ready to use.
6. Once the shrimp is done, carefully remove the toothpicks and transfer it to a serving plate.
7. Serve with white Keto sauce and Enjoy!

251. Roasted Chicken

Made for: dinner | **Prep Time:** 25 minutes | **Servings:** 04
Per Serving: Kcal: 553, Protein: 38g, Fat: 39g, Net Carb: 8g

INGREDIENTS

- ❖ Four chicken thighs
- ❖ 1½ pounds carrots, peeled and trimmed
- ❖ One large onion, peeled and cut into eighths
- ❖ One head of garlic

- ❖ Four tablespoons olive oil
- ❖ One tablespoon chopped fresh rosemary
- ❖ Kosher salt and freshly ground black pepper, to taste

INSTRUCTIONS

1. Preheat the oven to 425°F.
2. Arrange the carrots and onion in a single layer on a greased baking sheet.
3. Slice the top of a head of garlic; discard the top, and place it on the tray.
4. Drizzle 2 tablespoons of olive oil over the vegetables; season with the rosemary, and salt and pepper.
5. Top with the chicken thighs. Rub each leg with one teaspoon olive oil; season with salt and pepper.
6. Roast in the oven until the chicken skin is golden, and the carrots are tender, 15 to 20 minutes.
7. To serve, divide the vegetables and chicken thighs among four plates.

252. Crispy Keto Cauliflower

Made for: dinner | **Prep Time:** 10 minutes | **Servings:** 02
Per Serving: Kcal: 181, Protein: 15g, Fat: 12g, Net Carb: 4g

INGREDIENTS

- ❖ 2 large eggs.
- ❖ 12 oz cauliflower rice (frozen).
- ❖ Olive oil for frying.
- ❖ ½ cup (45g) parmesan (grated).
- ❖ ½ tsp salt.
- ❖ ¼ tsp black pepper.
- ❖ ⅛ tsp paprika.

INSTRUCTIONS

1. Microwave the cauliflower rice and allow it to soften.
2. Mix all ingredients, except the eggs, together with the rice until well combined.
3. When the mixture is thoroughly combined, stir in the eggs and mix well.
4. Heat olive oil in a large frying pan and scoop 1 heaped tbsp of mixture into the pan. Fry

for 2 minutes on each side until crispy and golden brown.
5. Repeat the process until all mixture has gone.

253. Peanut Butter Cookies

Prep Time: 20 minutes | **Servings:** 12 Cookies
Per Cookies: Kcal: 108, Protein: 5g, Fat: 9g, Net Carb: 4g

INGREDIENTS:

- ❖ 3/4 cup (190g) peanut butter
- ❖ 1/4 cup (25g) erythritol add more for sweeter cookies
- ❖ 1 large egg
- ❖ 2 tablespoons
- ❖ 1 tsp vanilla optional

INSTRUCTIONS

1. Pre-heat oven to 350F.
2. Add all the ingredients to a medium-large mixing bowl. Stir with a spatula until fully and mixed through. The batter will be runny at first and get harder as it is mixed.
3. Scoop out dough using a cookie scoop and shape it into a ball. Place on a baking sheet and flatten with a fork. Drizzle with salt if desired.
4. Bake 12 minutes. Cool for 10 minutes before serving.

254. Keto Everything Bagel

Made for: dinner | **Prep Time:** 20 minutes | **Servings:** 04
Per Serving: Kcal: 218, Protein: 14g, Fat: 17g, Net Carb: 3g

INGREDIENTS

- ❖ 1 cup (113g) shredded cheese, cheddar, mozzarella, any kind of cheese that melts well.
- ❖ ½ cup (45g) grated parmesan, or asiago, other hard, dry, grated cheese.
- ❖ 2 eggs
- ❖ 2 tbsp everything bagel seasoning

INSTRUCTIONS

1. Preheat oven to 375 degrees Fahrenheit.
2. Combine the shredded cheese and egg in a bowl and mix it until the ingredients are fully combined.
3. Divide the mixture equally into six parts and press into well greased donut pan.
4. Sprinkle everything bagel seasoning over the tops of the egg and cheese mixture.
5. Bake at 375 degrees for about 15 to 20 minutes until the cheese has fully melted and created a slight brown crust.
6. Feel free to mix up your cheese selection - but stick with one grated hard, dry cheese to keep the flour-like texture.

255. Bacon Cheeseburger Skillet

Made for: dinner | **Prep Time:** 25 minutes | **Servings:** 04
Per Serving: Kcal: 433, Protein: 9g, Fat: 13g, Net Carb: 3g

INGREDIENTS

- ❖ 4 slices of bacon, chopped into small pieces
- ❖ 1 pound of ground turkey or ground beef
- ❖ 1/2 cup (75g) chopped onion (about half of one small onion)
- ❖ 2 tablespoons tomato paste
- ❖ 1 teaspoon mustard
- ❖ 2 ounces cream cheese
- ❖ 1/2 cup (50g) chicken or beef broth
- ❖ 1/2 teaspoon onion powder
- ❖ 1/2 teaspoon garlic powder
- ❖ 1/4 teaspoon salt
- ❖ 1/4 teaspoon pepper
- ❖ 1 cup (110g) shredded cheddar cheese.

INSTRUCTIONS

1. Heat a large skillet over medium heat. Lightly spray with cooking spray.
2. Cook the chopped bacon until crisp and remove from the skillet and set aside.
3. Drain off all of the bacon grease except 1 tablespoon. Add the ground beef and onion. Brown the meat and drain off any grease.
4. Add the tomato paste, mustard, cream cheese, broth and spices stirring until the cream cheese has melted and a sauce has formed.

5. Reduce the heat to low and top with cooked bacon and remaining cheese.
6. Cover the skillet and cook on low for 5-7 minutes until cheese is completely melted.

256. Cheese & Tomato Salad

Made for: dinner | **Prep Time:** 10 minutes | **Servings:** 04
Per Serving: Kcal: 216, Protein: 15g, Fat: 18g, Net Carb: 3g

INGREDIENTS

- ❖ 8 oz mozzarella.
- ❖ 8 oz cherry tomatoes.
- ❖ 2 tbsp green pesto.

INSTRUCTIONS

1. Rip the mozzarella into bite-size pieces and halve the tomatoes.
2. Stir in the pesto until well combined.

257. Red Pepper and Basil

Made for: dinner | **Prep Time:** 25 minutes | **Servings:** 02
Per Serving: Kcal: 159, Protein: 4g, Fat: 8g, Net Carb: 5g

INGREDIENTS

- ❖ 2¼ pounds tomatoes, diced
- ❖ One red bell pepper, diced
- ❖ 1 European cucumber, peeled and diced
- ❖ One garlic clove
- ❖ One red onion, minced and divided
- ❖ Four tablespoons chopped basil, divided
- ❖ Kosher salt and freshly ground black pepper
- ❖ 2 cups (300g) cut cherry tomatoes
- ❖ Two tablespoons extra-virgin olive oil

INSTRUCTIONS

1. In a blender or the bowl of a food processor, combine the tomatoes, red bell pepper, cucumber, garlic, half of the red onion, and half of the basil. Puree the mixture until smooth.
2. Season the gazpacho with salt and pepper to taste and blend to combine.
3. Ladle the gazpacho into serving bowls and garnish with the remaining onion and basil,

the cherry tomatoes, and a small drizzle of olive oil. Serve immediately.

258. Citrus Salmon

Made for: dinner | **Prep Time:** 20 minutes | **Servings:** 04
Per Serving: Kcal: 224, Protein: 20g, Fat: 13g, Net Carb: 4g

INGREDIENTS

- ❖ Six orange slices
- ❖ Six lime slices
- ❖ Six salmon fillets (4 ounces each)
- ❖ 1 pound fresh asparagus, trimmed and halved
- ❖ Olive oil-flavoured cooking spray
- ❖ 1/2 teaspoon salt
- ❖ 1/4 teaspoon pepper
- ❖ Two tablespoons minced fresh parsley
- ❖ Three tablespoons lemon juice

INSTRUCTIONS

1. Preheat oven to 425°. Cut parchment or heavy-duty foil into six 15x10-in. Pieces; fold in half. Arrange citrus slices on one side of each piece. Top with fish and asparagus. Spritz with cooking spray. Sprinkle with salt, pepper, and parsley. Drizzle with lemon juice.
2. Fold parchment over fish; draw edges together and crimp with fingers to form tightly sealed packets. Place in baking pans.
3. Bake until fish flakes easily with a fork, 12-15 minutes. Open packets carefully to allow steam to escape.

259. Artichoke Chicken

Made for: dinner | **Prep Time:** 15 minutes | **Servings:** 04
Per Serving: Kcal: 228, Protein: 22g, Fat: 21g, Net Carb: 2g

INGREDIENTS

- ❖ Four boneless skinless chicken thighs (about 2 pounds)
- ❖ Two jars (7-1/2 ounces each) marinated quartered artichoke hearts, drained
- ❖ Two tablespoons olive oil
- ❖ One teaspoon salt
- ❖ 1/2 teaspoon pepper

- ❖ 1/4 cup shredded Parmesan cheese
- ❖ Two tablespoons minced fresh parsley

INSTRUCTIONS

1. Preheat broiler. In a large bowl, toss chicken and artichokes with oil, salt, and pepper. Transfer to a broiler pan.
2. Broil 3 in. From heat 8-10 minutes or until a thermometer inserted in chicken reads 170°, turning chicken and artichokes halfway through cooking. Sprinkle with cheese. Broil 1-2 minutes longer or until cheese is melted. Sprinkle with parsley.

260. Zucchini Noodles

Made for: dinner | **Prep Time:** 30 minutes | **Servings:** 02
Per Serving: Kcal: 203, Protein: 34g, Fat: 44g, Net Carb: 6g

INGREDIENTS

- ❖ Two large zucchini/Courgette (about 1-1/2 pounds)
- ❖ 1-1/2 teaspoons ground cumin
- ❖ 3/4 teaspoon salt, divided
- ❖ 1/2 teaspoon smoked paprika
- ❖ 1/2 teaspoon pepper
- ❖ 1/4 tsp garlic powder
- ❖ Four tilapia fillets (6 ounces each)
- ❖ Two teaspoons olive oil
- ❖ Two garlic cloves, minced
- ❖ 1 cup pico de gallo

INSTRUCTIONS

1. Trim ends of zucchini. Using a spiralizer, cut zucchini into thin strands.
2. Mix cumin, 1/2 teaspoon salt, smoked paprika, pepper, and garlic powder; sprinkle generously onto both sides of tilapia, in a large nonstick skillet, heat oil over medium-high heat. In batches, cook tilapia until fish just begins to flake easily with a fork, 2-3 minutes per side. Remove from pan; keep warm.
3. In the same pan, cook zucchini with garlic over medium-high heat until slightly softened, 1-2 minutes, continually tossing with tongs (do not overcook). Sprinkle with

remaining salt. Serve with tilapia and pico de gallo.

261. Keto Tuna Salad

Made for: dinner | **Prep Time:** 15 minutes | **Servings:** 04
Per Serving: Kcal: 146, Protein: 17g, Fat: 11g, Net Carb: 1g

INGREDIENTS

- ❖ 2 cans canned tuna fish, drained
- ❖ 3 Tbsp mayonnaise
- ❖ 2 Tbsp lemon juice
- ❖ 1 each minced green onion
- ❖ 1 each dill pickles

INSTRUCTIONS

1. On a cutting board, finely chop the green onion and pickle, transfer them to a bowl.
2. Open the tuna cans, and drain them of excess oil. Add the tuna to the bowl, along with the mayo and lemon juice.
3. Mix well using a fork. Add salt and pepper if desired.
4. You can eat it on its own, or serve it in lettuce cups.

262. Chicken & Goat Cheese

Made for: dinner | **Prep Time:** 20 minutes | **Servings:** 02
Per Serving: Kcal: 251, Protein: 29g, Fat: 11g, Net Carb: 4g

INGREDIENTS

- ❖ 1/2-pound boneless skinless chicken breasts, cut into 1-inch pieces
- ❖ 1/4 teaspoon salt
- ❖ 1/8 teaspoon pepper
- ❖ Two teaspoons olive oil
- ❖ 1 cup (175g) sliced fresh asparagus (1-inch pieces)
- ❖ One garlic clove, minced
- ❖ Three plum tomatoes, chopped
- ❖ Three tablespoons 2% milk
- ❖ Two tablespoons herbed fresh goat cheese, crumbled
- ❖ Hot cooked rice or pasta
- ❖ Additional goat cheese, optional

INSTRUCTIONS

1. Toss chicken with salt and pepper. In a large skillet, heat oil over medium-high heat; saute chicken until no longer pink, 4-6 minutes. Remove from pan; keep warm.
2. Add asparagus to skillet; cook and stir over medium-high heat 1 minute. Add garlic; cook and stir 30 seconds. Stir in tomatoes, milk, and two tablespoons cheese; cook, covered, over medium heat until cheese begins to melt, 2-3 minutes. Stir in chicken. Serve with rice. If desired, top with additional cheese.

263. Ginger Halibut with Brussels Sprouts

Made for: dinner | **Prep Time:** 25 minutes | **Servings:** 04
Per Serving: Kcal: 234, Protein: 24g, Fat: 12g, Net Carb: 7g

INGREDIENTS

- ❖ Four teaspoons lemon juice
- ❖ Four halibut fillets (4 to 6 ounces each)
- ❖ One teaspoon minced fresh ginger root
- ❖ 1/4 to 3/4 teaspoon salt, divided
- ❖ 1/4 teaspoon pepper
- ❖ 1/2 cup/125ml water
- ❖ 10 ounces (about 2-1/2 cups) fresh Brussels sprouts, halved
- ❖ Crushed red pepper flakes
- ❖ One tablespoon canola oil
- ❖ Five garlic cloves, sliced lengthwise
- ❖ Two tablespoons sesame oil
- ❖ Two tablespoons soy sauce
- ❖ Lemon slices, optional

INSTRUCTIONS

1. Brush lemon juice over halibut fillets. Sprinkle with minced ginger, 1/4 teaspoon salt, and pepper.
2. Place fish on an oiled grill rack, skin side down. Grill, covered, over medium heat (or broil 6 in. from heat) until fish just begins to flake easily with a fork, 6-8 minutes.
3. In a large skillet, bring water to a boil over medium-high heat. Add Brussels sprouts, pepper flakes, and, if desired, remaining salt.

Cook, covered, until tender, 5-7 minutes. Meanwhile, in a small skillet, heat oil over medium heat. Add garlic; cook until golden brown. Drain on paper towels.
4. Drizzle sesame oil and soy sauce over halibut. Serve with Brussels sprouts; sprinkle with fried garlic. If desired, serve with lemon slices.

264. Soy & butter salmon parcels

Made for: dinner | **Prep Time:** 30 minutes | **Servings:** 02
Per Serving: Kcal: 589, Protein: 36g, Fat: 43g, Net Carb: 5g

INGREDIENTS

- ❖ 2 tbsp butter
- ❖ 4 x 100g skinless salmon fillets
- ❖ 2 tbsp low-salt soy sauce
- ❖ 1 tbsp honey
- ❖ 1 tbsp sesame seeds
- ❖ 2 sliced spring onions
- ❖ For the cucumber salad
- ❖ 1 cucumber, finely sliced
- ❖ few drops sesame oil

INSTRUCTIONS

1. Heat the barbecue. If you are using coals, wait until they turn white. If you are indoors, heat a griddle pan. Cut four pieces of foil that will easily wrap a piece of salmon and lay them on the work surface. Spread a little butter onto the centre of each piece of foil to stop the salmon sticking. Lay the salmon on top. Mix the soy with the honey and divide it between the parcels, pouring it over the salmon. Dot any remaining butter on top and then fold the foil around the salmon tightly to make a parcel.
2. Put the parcels on the barbecue or griddle and cook for 5-10 mins. Check one parcel to see how it's getting along but be careful – it will be hot. Once the salmon is cooked, open the parcels and scatter some sesame and spring onion into each.
3. Mix the cucumber with a few drops of sesame oil and season with a little salt. Serve the salmon with the cucumber salad.

265. Mexican Cabbage Roll

Made for: dinner | Prep Time: 20 minutes | Servings: 04
Per Serving: Kcal: 186, Protein: 17g, Fat: 12g, Net Carb: 8g

INGREDIENTS

- 1 pound lean ground beef (90% lean)
- 1/2 teaspoon salt
- 3/4 teaspoon garlic powder
- 1/4 teaspoon pepper
- One tablespoon olive oil
- One medium onion, chopped
- 6 cups/540g chopped cabbage (about one small head)
- Three cans (4 ounces each) chopped green chiles
- 2 cups/500ml of water
- One can (14-1/2 ounces) reduced-sodium beef broth
- Two tablespoons minced fresh cilantro
- Optional toppings: pico de gallo and reduced-fat sour cream, optional

INSTRUCTIONS

1. In a large saucepan, cook and crumble beef with seasonings over medium-high heat until no longer pink, 5-7 minutes. Remove from pan.
2. In the same pan, heat oil over medium-high heat; saute onion and cabbage until crisp-tender, 4-6 minutes. Stir in beef, chiles, water, and broth; bring to a boil. Reduce heat; simmer, covered, to allow flavours to blend, about 10 minutes. Stir in cilantro. If desired, top with pico de gallo and sour cream.
3. Freeze option: Freeze cooled soup in freezer containers. To use, partially thaw in refrigerator overnight. Heat through in a saucepan, stirring occasionally.

266. Chicken Provolone

Made for: dinner | Prep Time: 25 minutes | Servings: 04
Per Serving: Kcal: 236, Protein: 33g, Fat: 12g, Net Carb: 2g

INGREDIENTS

- Four boneless skinless chicken breast halves (4 ounces each)
- 1/4 teaspoon pepper
- Eight fresh basil leaves
- Butter-flavoured cooking spray
- Four thin slices prosciutto or deli ham
- 4 slices provolone cheese

INSTRUCTIONS

1. Sprinkle chicken with pepper. In a large skillet coated with cooking spray, cook chicken over medium heat until a thermometer reads 165°, 4-5 minutes on each side.
2. Transfer to an ungreased baking sheet; top with the basil, prosciutto, and cheese. Broil 6-8 in. From the heat until cheese is melted, 1-2 minutes.

267. Lemon-Pepper Tilapia

Made for: dinner | Prep Time: 20 minutes | Servings: 04
Per Serving: Kcal: 216, Protein: 34g, Fat: 8g, Net Carb: 5g

INGREDIENTS

- Two tablespoons butter
- 1/2 pound sliced fresh mushrooms
- 3/4 teaspoon lemon-pepper seasoning, divided
- Three garlic cloves, minced
- Four tilapia fillets (6 ounces each)
- 1/4 teaspoon paprika
- 1/8 teaspoon cayenne pepper
- One medium tomato, chopped
- Three green onions, thinly sliced

INSTRUCTIONS

1. In a 12-in. Skillet, heat butter over medium heat. Add mushrooms and 1/4 teaspoon lemon pepper; cook and stir 3-5 minutes or until tender. Add garlic; cook 30 seconds longer.
2. Place fillets over mushrooms; sprinkle with paprika, cayenne, and remaining lemon pepper. Cook, covered, 5-7 minutes or until fish just begins to flake easily with a fork. Top with tomato and green onions.

268. Bountiful Bacon, Cheese

Made for: dinner | **Prep Time:** 30 minutes | **Servings:** 02
Per Serving: Kcal: 273, Protein: 9g, Fat: 29g, Net Carb: 2g

INGREDIENTS

- ❖ 5 oz cheddar cheese (grated).
- ❖ 5 oz cream cheese.
- ❖ 5 oz bacon.
- ❖ 2 oz butter.
- ❖ ½ tsp chilli flakes.
- ❖ ½ tsp black pepper.
- ❖ ½ tsp Italian seasoning.

INSTRUCTIONS

1. Heat the butter in a large frying pan and fry the bacon until crispy. Reserve bacon fat and chop the bacon into small pieces.
2. In a bowl, mix cream cheese, cheddar cheese, chilli flakes, pepper, Italian seasoning, and bacon fat until well combined.
3. Place the cream cheese mix in the fridge for 20 minutes.
4. When the mixture is set, roll 24 balls into shape.
5. Roll each ball in the bacon pieces before serving.

269. Sensational Smoked

Made for: dinner | **Prep Time:** 25 minutes | **Servings:** 02
Per Serving: Kcal: 255, Protein: 10g, Fat: 20g, Net Carb: 3g

INGREDIENTS

- ❖ 4 oz cream cheese
- ❖ 3 oz smoked salmon (canned and drained).
- ❖ 1 oz iceberg lettuce leaves.
- ❖ 3 tbsp mayonnaise.
- ❖ 2 tbsp chives (finely chopped).
- ❖ ½ lemon zest.

INSTRUCTIONS

1. In a large bowl, mix everything (except lettuce leaves) together until well combined.
2. Place in the refrigerator for 15-20 minutes.

3. When chilled, scoop onto lettuce leaves and serve.

270. Zucchini Noodles

Made for: dinner | **Prep Time:** 25 minutes | **Servings:** 02
Per Serving: Kcal: 801, Protein: 21g, Fat: 78g, Net Carb: 6g

INGREDIENTS

- ❖ 16 oz zucchini/Courgette.
- ❖ 5 oz bacon (diced).
- ❖ One ¼ cups thick double cream.
- ❖ ¼ cup (60g) mayonnaise.
- ❖ 2 oz parmesan (grated).
- ❖ 1 tbsp butter.

INSTRUCTIONS

1. Heat the cream in a large saucepan; bring to a gentle boil and allow to reduce slightly.
2. Heat the butter in a large frying pan and cook the bacon until crispy; set aside and leave grease warming in the pan (low heat).
3. Add the mayonnaise to the cream and turn down the heat.
4. Using a potato peeler, make thin zucchini strips—Cook the zucchini noodles for 30 seconds in a pan of boiling water.
5. Add cream mixture and bacon fat to the zucchini noodles, tossing to ensure all are coated. Mix in the bacon and parmesan

271. Tuna Burgers on a Bed

Made for: dinner | **Prep Time:** 15 minutes | **Servings:** 02
Per Serving: Kcal: 250, Protein: 21g, Fat: 16g, Net Carb: 2g

INGREDIENTS

- ❖ 16 oz tinned tuna (drained).
- ❖ 8 oz baby spinach.
- ❖ Two onions (finely diced).
- ❖ One large egg.
- ❖ ¼ cup/60 mayonnaise.
- ❖ ⅓ cup/38g almond flour.
- ❖ 2 tbsp fresh dill (finely chopped).
- ❖ 1 tbsp lemon zest.
- ❖ 1 tbsp olive oil.
- ❖ 2 tbsp avocado oil.

INSTRUCTIONS

1. In a large bowl, mix tuna, onions, egg, mayonnaise, almond flour, dill, and lemon zest.
2. From the mixture, form 8 burgers.
3. Heat 1 tbsp avocado oil in a large frying pan, fry four tuna patties for 4-5 minutes, flip and cook for an additional 4 minutes. Repeat with remaining oil and burgers.
4. Place the spinach on a serving plate and drizzle with olive oil, top with burgers.

272. Salmon & Creamy Spinach

Made for: dinner | **Prep Time:** 25 minutes | **Servings:** 04
Per Serving: Kcal: 667, Protein: 54g, Fat: 38g, Net Carb: 5g

INGREDIENTS

- ❖ 10 oz tinned salmon.
- ❖ 9 oz spinach (frozen).
- ❖ 1 ½ cups/135g parmesan (grated).
- ❖ One cup/232g of thick cream/single cream
- ❖ ½ cup/130ml of almond milk.
- ❖ ¼ cup/55g butter.
- ❖ Four slices mozzarella.
- ❖ One garlic clove (crushed).
- ❖ 1 tbsp parsley (dried).

INSTRUCTIONS

1. Preheat the oven at 180 degrees.
2. In a large saucepan, heat the butter with the garlic. When garlic is browned, add in almond milk and cream.
3. Heat for 5-6 minutes and stir in parmesan, spinach, parsley, and salmon.
4. Continuously stir until the mixture is bubbling...
5. Pour into an ovenproof dish and top with mozzarella cheese.
6. Bake for 25-30 minutes until bubbling and golden.

273. California Burger Wraps

Made for: dinner | **Prep Time:** 30 minutes | **Servings:** 04
Per Serving: Kcal: 252, Protein: 24g, Fat: 15g, Net Carb: 6g

INGREDIENTS

- ❖ 1-pound lean ground beef (90% lean)
- ❖ 1/2 teaspoon salt
- ❖ 1/4 teaspoon pepper
- ❖ 8 Bibb lettuce leaves
- ❖ 1/3 cup/50g crumbled feta cheese
- ❖ Two tablespoons Miracle Whip Light
- ❖ 1/2 medium ripe avocado, peeled and cut into eight slices
- ❖ 1/4 cup/38g chopped red onion
- ❖ Chopped cherry tomatoes, optional

INSTRUCTIONS

1. In a large bowl, combine beef, salt, and pepper, mixing lightly but thoroughly. Shape into eight 1/2-in.-thick patties.
2. Grill burgers, covered, over medium heat or broil 3-4 in. From heat until a thermometer reads 160°, 3-4 minutes on each side. Place burgers in lettuce leaves. Combine feta and Miracle Whip; spread over burgers. Top with avocado, red onion, and if desired, tomatoes.

274. Chicken & pistachio salad

Made for: dinner | **Prep Time:** 15 minutes | **Servings:** 02
Per Serving: Kcal: 521, Protein: 37g, Fat: 30g, Net Carb: 2g

INGREDIENTS

- ❖ 2 large eggs
- ❖ 2 tbsp extra virgin olive oil
- ❖ 1 large lemon, zested and juiced
- ❖ 2 tbsp natural yogurt
- ❖ 1 large skinless cooked chicken breast fillet
- ❖ 40g (1/8 cup) mixed olives, halved
- ❖ 40g (1/3 cup) sundried tomatoes
- ❖ small bunch basil, chopped
- ❖ 3 Little Gem lettuces, leaves separated
- ❖ 30g (1/4 cup) pistachios, roughly chopped and toasted

INSTRUCTIONS

1. Bring a large pan of water to a simmer. Add the eggs and cook gently for 7 mins. Remove with a slotted spoon and transfer to a bowl

of cold water. Once cooled, carefully peel off the shell and slice each egg in half.
2. Meanwhile, whisk the oil with the lemon zest, juice and yogurt, and season well. Shred the chicken and toss with the olives, sundried tomatoes, basil and lettuce. Pour in the dressing, season and toss together.
3. Divide the salad between two bowls and top with the egg halves and pistachios.

275. Chicken Nicoise Salad

Made for: dinner | **Prep Time:** 20 minutes | **Servings:** 02
Per Serving: Kcal: 289, Protein: 24g, Fat: 18g, Net Carb: 4g

INGREDIENTS

❖ 1/2-pound fresh green beans, trimmed and halved (about 1 cup)
   DRESSING:
❖ 1/4 cup/60ml olive oil
❖ Two teaspoons grated lemon zest
❖ Two tablespoons lemon juice
❖ Two garlic cloves, minced
❖ One teaspoon Dijon mustard
❖ 1/8 teaspoon salt
❖ Dash pepper

SALAD:

❖ One can (5 ounces) light tuna in water, drained and flaked
❖ Two tablespoons sliced ripe olives, drained
❖ One teaspoon caper, rinsed and drained
❖ 2 cups torn mixed salad greens
❖ One package (6 ounces) ready-to-use Southwest-style grilled chicken breast strips
❖ One small red onion halved and thinly sliced
❖ One medium sweet red pepper, julienned
❖ Two large hard-boiled eggs, cut into wedges

INSTRUCTIONS

1. In a saucepan, cook green beans in boiling water just until crisp-tender. Remove and immediately drop into ice water to cool. Drain; pat dry.
2. Meanwhile, whisk together dressing ingredients. In a small bowl, lightly toss tuna with olives and capers.

3. Line platter with salad greens; top with tuna mixture, green beans, and remaining ingredients. Serve with dressing.

276. Cauliflower & Ham Bake

Made for: dinner | **Prep Time:** 25 minutes | **Servings:** 02
Per Serving: Kcal: 447, Protein: 42g, Fat: 21g, Net Carb: 8g

INGREDIENTS

❖ 2 large eggs.
❖ Two garlic cloves (crushed).
❖ ⅔ cup/160ml of almond milk (unsweetened).
❖ ½ cup/100ml of dry white wine.
❖ ½ cup/55g cheddar cheese (grated).
❖ ½ cup/55g mozzarella (grated).
❖ 10 oz spinach (frozen & defrosted).
❖ 8 oz cooked ham.
❖ 1 tbsp olive oil.

INSTRUCTIONS

1. Preheat the oven at 190 degrees.
2. In a large bowl, mix spinach, cauliflower rice, milk, eggs, ⅓ cup mozzarella, and ⅓ cup cheddar.
3. In a large frying pan, heat the olive oil and fry the garlic until lightly browned. Stir in the white wine and cook until wine evaporates; add the ham and cook for 2-3 minutes.
4. Combine the ham mixture to the spinach mixture.
5. Add mixture to an ovenproof dish, sprinkle the remaining cheese on top.
6. Bake for 30-35 minutes until golden brown.

277. Moroccan Cauliflower

Made for: dinner | **Prep Time:** 25 minutes | **Servings:** 02
Per Serving: Kcal: 150, Protein: 12g, Fat: 23g, Net Carb: 8g

INGREDIENTS

❖ One large head cauliflower (about 3-1/2 pounds), broken into florets
❖ 6 cups vegetable stock
❖ 3/4 cup/70g sliced almonds, toasted iand divided

- 1/2 cup/8g plus two tablespoons minced fresh cilantro, divided
- Two tablespoons olive oil
- 1 to 3 teaspoons harissa chilli paste or hot pepper sauce
- 1/2 teaspoon ground cinnamon
- 1/2 teaspoon ground cumin
- 1/2 teaspoon ground coriander
- 1-1/4 teaspoons salt
- 1/2 teaspoon pepper
- Additional harissa chilli paste, optional

INSTRUCTIONS

1. In a 5- or 6-qt. Slow cooker, combine cauliflower, vegetable stock, 1/2 cup almonds, 1/2 cup cilantro, and the next seven ingredients. Cook, covered, on low until cauliflower is tender, 6-8 hours.
2. Puree soup using an immersion blender. Or cool slightly and puree the soup in batches in a blender; return to slow cooker and heat through. Serve with remaining almonds and cilantro and, if desired, additional harissa.

278. Coconut Bed of Buttered

Made for: dinner | **Prep Time:** 25 minutes | **Servings:** 02
Per Serving: Kcal: 768, Protein: 33g, Fat: 69g, Net Carb: 3g

INGREDIENTS

- 8 oz salmon fillets (frozen & defrosted).
- 8 oz white cabbage.
- 2 oz butter.
- 1 oz shredded coconut (unsweetened).
- 3 tbsp olive oil.
- 1 tsp turmeric.
- ½ tsp onion powder.

INSTRUCTIONS

1. Cut the salmon into bite-size pieces and drizzle over olive oil.
2. In a small bowl, mix coconut, turmeric, and onion powder. Dip each salmon chunk into the coconut mix until the salmon is well coated.
3. In a frying pan, fry the salmon until golden brown; cover with foil and set aside.

4. Melt the butter in the frying pan and fry the cabbage until it begins to lightly brown.
5. Place the cabbage on a plate and the salmon on top; drizzle with olive oil.

279. Cheese Pancakes

Made for: dinner | **Prep Time:** 20 minutes | **Servings:** 02
Per Serving: Kcal: 651, Protein: 31g, Fat: 59g, Net Carb: 5g

INGREDIENTS

- 4 ounces cream cheese, at room temperature
- 2 large eggs
- 1/4 cup/28g flour, such as almond, coconut, or all-purpose
- 1/2 teaspoon baking powder
- 1/4 teaspoon fine salt
- Cooking spray or butter, for greasing the pan
- Sliced strawberries and powdered sugar, or maple syrup, for serving

INSTRUCTIONS

1. Place the cream cheese, eggs, flour, baking powder, and salt in a blender and blend until smooth.
2. Heat a large nonstick frying pan over medium heat. Coat with cooking spray or butter. Once the butter is melted, pour in 2 to 3 tablespoons of the batter. Cook until deep golden-brown on the bottom, about 3 minutes. Flip and cook until the second side is golden-brown, 1 to 2 minutes more. Transfer to a plate.
3. Repeat with cooking remaining batter. Serve with sliced strawberries and powdered sugar.

280. Butternut Squash

Made for: dinner | **Prep Time:** 35 minutes | **Servings:** 02
Per Serving: Kcal: 325, Protein: 19g, Fat: 10g, Net Carb: 4g

INGREDIENTS

- ❖ One medium butternut squash (about 3 pounds)
- ❖ 1 pound Italian turkey sausage links, casings removed
- ❖ One medium onion, finely chopped
- ❖ Four garlic cloves, minced
- ❖ 1/2 cup (55g) shredded Italian cheese blend
- ❖ Crushed red pepper flakes, optional

INSTRUCTIONS

1. Preheat broiler. Cut squash lengthwise in half; discard seeds. Place squash in a large microwave-safe dish, cut side down; add 1/2 in. Of water. Microwave, covered, on high until soft, 20-25 minutes. Cool slightly.
2. Meanwhile, in a large nonstick skillet, cook and crumble sausage with onion over medium-high heat until no longer pink, 5-7 minutes. Add garlic; cook and stir 1 minute.
3. Leaving 1/2-in.-thick shells, scoop pulp from the squash and stir into sausage mixture. Place squash shells on a baking sheet; fill with sausage mixture. Sprinkle with cheese.
4. Broil 4-5 in. From heat until cheese is melted, 1-2 minutes. If desired, sprinkle with pepper flakes. To serve, cut each half into two portions.

Keto Vegitarian Recipes

281. Broccoli Cheese Bites

Prep Time: 25 minutes | **Servings:** 24 bites
Per Bites: Kcal: 23, Protein: 1g, Fat: 1g, Net Carb: 1g

INGREDIENTS

- ❖ 2 heads Broccoli
- ❖ 1/2 cup (75g) frozen spinach defrosted and drained well
- ❖ 1/4 cup (25g) Scallions sliced
- ❖ 1 Lemon Zest only
- ❖ 1 cup (110g) Cheddar Cheese grated
- ❖ 1/4 cup (90g) Parmesan cheese grated
- ❖ 2 eggs
- ❖ 1/3 cup (80g) Sour Cream

- ❖ 1/2 teaspoon Pepper
- ❖ 1/4 teaspoon Salt

INSTRUCTIONS

1. Preheat oven to 180C/355F.
2. Cut broccoli into evenly sized florets and place in a microwave safe container with ¼ cup of water. Microwave on high for 3 minutes or until the broccoli is tender. Drain well and allow to cool.
3. Chop the broccoli into very small pieces, You should end up with approximately 2-2 ½ cups.
4. Place the chopped broccoli in a bowl with all the remaining ingredients and mix well.
5. Pour the mixture into a 11 x 7in rectangle brownie pan, lined with parchment paper, and smooth into an even layer.
6. Bake for 25 minutes, until the bites are puffed and browning.
7. Allow to cool for 10 minutes, before cutting into 24 squares.

282. Keto Vegetable Bake

Prep Time: 35 minutes | **Servings:** 4
Per Servings: Kcal: 260, Protein: 8g, Fat: 20g, Net Carb: 2g

INGREDIENTS

- ❖ 1 zucchini/courgette
- ❖ 1 red capsicum
- ❖ 1/2 red onion
- ❖ 1 head of broccoli

    Sauce
- ❖ 1/2 cup (125g) pesto
- ❖ 1/4 cup (60g) cream
- ❖ 4 tablespoons parmesan cheese
- ❖ 1/4 teaspoon salt
- ❖ Fresh basil or celery leaves to serve

INSTRUCTIONS

1. Preheat the oven to 180C/356F and grease a small baking dish
2. Chop the vegetables into rough chunks and the onion into small wedges, separating the layers.

3. Combine the sauce ingredients and toss through the chopped vegetables and pour into the baking dish.
4. Bake for 30 minutes, stirring halfway through and serve warm with fresh basil

283. Easy Cheesy Zucchini

Prep Time: 45 minutes | Servings: 04
Per Servings: Kcal: 230, Protein: 8g, Fat: 20g, Net Carb: 3g

INGREDIENTS

- ❖ 4 cups (450g) sliced raw zucchini/Courgette
- ❖ 1 small onion, peeled and sliced thin
- ❖ salt and pepper to taste
- ❖ 1 1/2 cups (175g) shredded pepper jack cheese
- ❖ 2 Tbsp butter
- ❖ 1/2 tsp garlic powder
- ❖ 1/2 cup (120ml) heavy whipping cream/double cream
- ❖ 1/4 teaspoon xanthan gum

INSTRUCTIONS

1. Preheat oven to 375 degrees (F).
2. Grease a 9×9 or equivalent oven proof pan.
3. Overlap 1/3 of the zucchini and onion slices in the pan, then season with salt and pepper and sprinkle with 1/2 cup of shredded cheese.
4. Repeat two more times until you have three layers and have used up all of the zucchini, onions, and shredded cheese.
5. Combine the garlic powder, butter, heavy cream, and xanthan gum in a microwave safe dish.
6. Heat for one minute or until the butter has melted. Whisk until smooth.
7. Gently pour the butter and cream mixture over the zucchini layers.
8. Bake at 375 degrees (F) for about 45 minutes, or until the liquid has thickened and the top is golden brown.
9. Serve warm.

284. Low-Carb Spinach

Prep Time: 35 minutes | Servings: 02
Per Servings: Kcal: 198, Protein: 20g, Fat: 23g, Net Carb: 4g

INGREDIENTS

- ❖ 8.8 oz spinach (8.8 oz = 250g) (if frozen, let defrost)
- ❖ 5 eggs
- ❖ 1.5 cup/180g cheddar cheese
- ❖ 2 tomatoes
- ❖ ½ tsp garlic powder (or garlic salt)
- ❖ 1 tsp nutmeg
- ❖ 1 tsp onion powder
- ❖ 1 tbsp basil (dried is also fine)
- ❖ 1 tbsp oregano (dried is also fine)
- ❖ Salt and pepper to taste
- ❖ 1 tbsp olive oil (for greasing the tray)

INSTRUCTIONS

1. Preheat the oven to 200°C/390°F.
2. Beat the eggs in a large bowl.
3. Add the garlic, nutmeg, onion powder, salt and pepper.
4. Grate the cheese.
5. Give it all a stir then mix in the spinach and cheese.
6. Make sure everything is thoroughly coated in egg and spice mix.
7. Pour into a 9 inch pie tin (grease with a little oil first), spread it evenly and get it in the oven!
8. Slice the tomatoes.
9. After about 20 minutes of cooking, take out the pie and layer the tomatoes on top.
10. Cook for another 15-20 mins.
11. When ready, sprinkle on the basil, oregano and a little more salt and pepper.
12. Done! Serve, and enjoy.

285. Keto Vegetable Soup

Prep Time: 45 minutes | Servings: 04
Per Servings: Kcal: 130, Protein: 8g, Fat: 39g, Net Carb: 3g

INGREDIENTS

- ❖ 1/2 tablespoon butter

- ❖ 1/2 tablespoon olive oil
- ❖ 1/2 medium onion, chopped
- ❖ 1 stalk celery, chopped
- ❖ 1 carrot, peeled and chopped
- ❖ 2 cloves garlic, minced
- ❖ 1 cup/115g chopped cauliflower florets
- ❖ 1 cup/150g fresh green beans, trimmed and cut into 1-inch pieces
- ❖ 30 ounces canned diced tomatoes
- ❖ 4 cups/960g beef broth
- ❖ 1/2 tablespoon Worcestershire sauce
- ❖ 1/2 tablespoon Italian seasoning
- ❖ 1/2 teaspoon salt
- ❖ 1/2 teaspoon cracked pepper
- ❖ 1 cup/30g fresh spinach

INSTRUCTIONS

1. Add the butter and olive to a large stock pot over medium heat until butter has melted.
2. Add the onions, celery, carrots, and garlic and cook for 5 minutes, stirring often.
3. Add the cauliflower, green beans, tomatoes, beef broth, Worcestershire sauce, and Italian seasoning. Stir to combine.
4. Bring to a boil, reduce to a simmer, and cook for 25 minutes or until vegetable are tender.
5. Season with the salt and pepper and add the spinach to the pot. Stir well and continue cooking for 1-2 minutes until the spinach has wilted.
6. Taste and add additional salt and pepper, if needed. Serve immediately.

286. Roasted Veggies

Prep Time: 35 minutes | **Servings:** 10
Per Servings: Kcal: 55, Protein: 2g, Fat: 3g, Net Carb: 2g

INGREDIENTS

- ❖ 1 ½ cups (115g) radishes
- ❖ 1 ½ cups (125g) Brussels sprouts
- ❖ 1 yellow squash
- ❖ 1 zucchini/Courgette
- ❖ 1 Red pepper
- ❖ 1 Yellow Pepper
- ❖ Salt and pepper to taste
- ❖ 1 tsp. Oregano
- ❖ 1 tsp basil

- ❖ 1 tsp parsley
- ❖ 1 Tbsp Coconut oil, melted

INSTRUCTIONS

1. Preheat the oven to 425°F.
2. Wash all veggies well first, peel the zucchini and squash first if you like.
3. Rough chop everything into bite size pieces, in general I cut brussel sprouts and radishes in half unless they were very large. These take longer to cook and will cook more evenly in smaller pieces.
4. In a large bowl toss together the chopped veggies, coconut oil, and herbs until all vegetables are well coated in oil and seasoning.
5. Spread vegetables out as much as you can over a large baking sheet, drizzle a little more oil on them if they are not wet enough, healthy oils are our friend.
6. Salt and pepper to taste, I like to use a fresh ground black pepper and coarse ground sea salt when roasting veggies to really bring out the flavors.
7. Let your vegetables roast for 20-30 minutes, depending on how softened and browned you like them. I like to leave mine in longer and get that delicious caramelized flavor and char on the tips.
8. Remove from oven and serve with your favorite protein and healthy fats for a tasty and pretty meal!

287. Roasted Vegetable Salad

Prep Time: 15 minutes | **Servings:** 04
Per Servings: Kcal: 150, Protein: 16g, Fat: 65g, Net Carb: 3g

INGREDIENTS

- ❖ 1 Red Bell Pepper
- ❖ 1 Green Bell Pepper
- ❖ 1 Yellow Bell Pepper
- ❖ ½ of Head Cauliflower
- ❖ ¾ Cup (100g) Diced Cucumber
- ❖ ½ Cup (75g) Feta (crumbled)
- ❖ 1½ Tbsp Olive Oil
- ❖ Salt and Pepper (to taste)
- ❖ 2 Tbsp Balsamic Salad Dressing

- ❖ ¼ Cup (5g) Fresh Basil (chopped)
- ❖ ¼ Cup (15g) Fresh Parsley (chopped)

INSTRUCTIONS

1. Preheat your bbq or oven to 400 F. (if your bbq doesn't have a thermometer, just preheat it on medium low heat for 4 - 5 minutes)
2. Chop the peppers and cauliflower into 1 inch pieces. Place the vegetables into a mixing bowl and drizzle with the olive oil. Season with salt and pepper, then mix until the vegetables are fully coated in the oil. Spread the veggies onto a cookie sheet or bbq safe roasting pan.
3. Place the pan onto the top rack of your bbq or into a preheated oven. Roast the vegetables for 7 - 8 minutes or just until tender. Remove from the heat and let cool completely. (Once the veggies have cooled enough... put them into the refrigerator)
4. Dice up the cucumber and chop the fresh herbs. Add both to the mixing bowl with the cooled vegetables. Then cover with the balsamic dressing and feta cheese. Mix until the salad is fully coated in the dressing. Garnish with a piece of fresh parsley or basil.

288. Loaded Cauliflower

Prep Time: 25 minutes | **Servings:** 04
Per Servings: Kcal: 170, Protein: 8g, Fat: 15g, Net Carb: 3g

INGREDIENTS

- ❖ 1 head cauliflower (steamed) or 6 cups Steamed Cauliflower Rice
- ❖ 1 cup (112g) shredded cheddar cheese, divided
- ❖ 1/2 cup (120g) sour cream
- ❖ 2 teaspoons dry ranch seasoning
- ❖ 1 teaspoon onion powder
- ❖ 1 teaspoon garlic powder
- ❖ 4 tablespoons real bacon bits, divided

INSTRUCTIONS

1. preheat oven to 350

2. You need to first steam your fresh cauliflower head. Break apart the head of the cauliflower and discard the green leaves. Steam cauliflower until a fork can easily be stuck into the vegetable. Mash cauliflower in a large mixing bowl. Season with salt and pepper.
3. If you prefer to use cauliflower rice, you need approximately 6 cups of steamed cauliflower rice.
4. Set aside 1 tablespoon shredded cheddar cheese and then add remaining cheddar cheese, sour cream, ranch seasoning, onion powder, garlic powder and 3 tablespoons of bacon bits to the cauliflower and mix well. If you are adding whole whipping cream as the optional ingredient, add at this stage.
5. Transfer cauliflower into a small baking dish and heat for 35 minutes until hot.
6. Remove from oven and immediately sprinkle with remaining cheddar cheese and 1 tablespoon bacon bits.
7. Serve white hot and melty.

289. Bacon Butter Roasted

Prep Time: 30 minutes | **Servings:** 02
Per Servings: Kcal: 350, Protein: 20g, Fat: 28g, Net Carb: 4g

INGREDIENTS

- ❖ 1/2 lb (250g) bacon, cooked crispy and chopped
- ❖ 2 pounds brussel sprouts, trimmed and sliced into thirds
- ❖ 1 head cauliflower, heart removed and florets sliced
- ❖ 4 tbsp butter, softened
- ❖ 2 tbsp olive oil
- ❖ 2 garlic cloves, minced
- ❖ 1/2 lemon, for juice and zest
- ❖ Pepper (salt optional, we did not use it because of the bacon)

INSTRUCTIONS

1. Preheat oven to 375
2. In a large bowl, toss veggies, olive oil, pepper and 1 big squeeze of lemon together

until evenly coated. Set aside

3. In a small bowl, smash and mix softened butter until it is smooth. Stir in 1/2 cup of crumbled, chopped bacon and continue mixing.
4. Add veggies to a sheet pan, top with remaining bacon
5. Place little pats of the bacon butter over the top evenly. You may have leftover butter. We only used about 2 tbsp equivalent.
6. Roast for 25-30 mins, turning and mixing half way through.
7. Finish with lemon zest before serving.

290. Keto Stir Fry

Prep Time: 35 minutes | **Servings:** 02
Per Servings: Kcal: 250, Protein: 20g, Fat: 23g, Net Carb: 1g

INGREDIENTS

Stir Fry
- ❖ 4 tbsp olive oil
- ❖ 1 lb shrimp
- ❖ 8 cups vegetables, in bite-sized pieces/slices (see notes below)

Sauce
- ❖ 1 tsp ginger paste
- ❖ 2 tsp garlic
- ❖ 1/4 cup/60g coconut or liquid aminos, tamari sauce, or soy
- ❖ 4 tsp sesame oil
- ❖ 1/8 to 1/4 tsp red pepper flakes
- ❖ 1/2 tsp xantham gum (or, 2 tsp cornstarch if not following keto)

INSTRUCTIONS

1. In a small bowl, whisk together ginger paste, garlic, coconut aminos, sesame oil, red pepper flakes, and xantham gum. Set aside
2. Heat oil in a skillet or wok until very hot (but not smoking), add shrimp and saute until pink. Remove shrimp from pan, cover with foil and keep warm.
3. Add broccoli and carrots. Saute for 3 minutes, stirring frequently.

4. Add zucchini, bell peppers, and mushrooms. Saute for 3 minutes stirring frequently.
5. Add cabbage and green onion. Saute for 2 minutes. Test veggies for doneness. If needed, continue sauteing until veggies are done to your likeness.
6. Add shrimp back to the pan and stir all together.
7. Pour sauce over veggies and shrimp and stir for 1 minute.
8. Remove from heat and serve!

291. Keto Tzatziki

Prep Time: 30 minutes | **Servings:** 04
Per Servings: Kcal: 200, Protein: 6g, Fat: 20g, Net Carb: 1g

INGREDIENTS

- ❖ 1 english cucumber, seeded and finely diced
- ❖ 1 ⅓ cups/340g greek yogurt
- ❖ 4 tbsp olive oil
- ❖ 1 tbsp lemon juice
- ❖ 2 tbsp fresh dill, chopped
- ❖ 2 tbsp minced garlic
- ❖ 1 tsp sea salt
- ❖ 1 tsp pepper

INSTRUCTIONS

1. Slice and seed the cucumber, finely chop.
2. Combine all ingredients and mix well.
3. Allow the dip to chill overnight for best flavor.

292. Cheese Pancakes

Prep Time: 10 minutes | **Servings:** 02
Per Servings: Kcal: 322, Protein: 11g, Fat: 31g, Net Carb: 1g

INGREDIENTS

- ❖ ½ tbsp butter
- ❖ 2 eggs
- ❖ 3/5 cup cream cheese (3/5 cup = 2.5oz)

INSTRUCTIONS

1. Add some butter to a pan and stick it on medium heat.

2. Throw the cream cheese and eggs into a bowl and mix with a fork until creamy. If you're planning to, now is the time to add some extras. But be careful! The batter is quite runny, so I wouldn't add things like nuts.
3. Alternatively, you can use a, but remember to let the batter sit for a minute or two! It'll cook better then.
4. Off it goes into the pan. I usually make just one big pancake, but two medium-sized ones would also work perfectly fine.
5. Enjoy!

293. Spinach and Cheese Pie

Prep Time: 40 minutes | Servings: 04
Per Servings: Kcal: 320, Protein: 21g, Fat: 23g, Net Carb: 1g

INGREDIENTS

- ❖ 8.8 oz spinach (8.8 oz = 250g) (if frozen, let defrost)
- ❖ 5 eggs
- ❖ 1.5 cup cheddar cheese (1.5 cup = 185g)
- ❖ 2 tomatoes
- ❖ ½ tsp garlic powder (or garlic salt)
- ❖ 1 tsp nutmeg
- ❖ 1 tsp onion powder
- ❖ 1 tbsp basil (dried is also fine)
- ❖ 1 tbsp oregano (dried is also fine)
- ❖ Salt and pepper to taste
- ❖ 1 tbsp olive oil (for greasing the tray)

INSTRUCTIONS

1. Preheat the oven to 200°C/390°F.
2. Beat the eggs in ia large bowl.
3. Add the garlic, nutmeg, onion powder, salt and pepper.
4. Grate the cheese.
5. Give it all a stir then mix in the spinach and cheese.
6. Make sure everything is thoroughly coated in egg and spice mix.
7. Pour into a 9-inch pie tin (grease with a little oil first), spread it evenly and get it in the oven!
8. Slice the tomatoes.

9. After about 20 minutes of cooking, take out the pie and layer the tomatoes on top.
10. Cook for another 15-20 mins.
11. When ready, sprinkle on the basil, oregano and a little more salt and pepper.
12. Done! Serve, and enjoy.

294. Vegan Keto Breakfast

Prep Time: 15 minutes | Servings: 01
Per Servings: Kcal: 152, Protein: 5g, Fat: 11g, Net Carb: 2g

INGREDIENTS

- ❖ 50g frozen berries (strawberry, raspberry, blueberry, blackberry – or a mix of them)
- ❖ 200g Alpro soy yogurt with coconut (or plain)
- ❖ 1/2 tsp cinnamon
- ❖ optional 1/4 tsp stevia (if you like it extra sweet – I used Natvia)
- ❖ 30g Pip & Nut almond & coconut butter (a dream!)
- ❖ 1 tsp cacao nibs

INSTRUCTIONS

1. Add the frozen berries, cinnamon and stevia to a large container and add the yogurt on top.
2. Using a stick blender combine all ingredients. I figured a stick blender works best for me as it is quite a small amount for a regular blender size.
3. Add to a bowl, top with the almond & coconut butter and cacao and voila: breakfast is served!
4. Are you looking for more keto recipes? Get in touch and let me know whether you're after more snacks, breakfasts or mains and I'll happily include more on the blog.

295. Keto Butter Cauliflower

Prep Time: 35 minutes | Servings: 02
Per Servings: Kcal: 475, Protein: 8g, Fat: 55g, Net Carb: 1g

INGREDIENTS

- ❖ 400g (1 lb) cauliflower

- ❖ 400ml canned full-fat coconut milk
- ❖ 30 g shallot (or white onion)
- ❖ 2 1/2 tbsp extra virgin olive oil
- ❖ 1 tbsp coconut oil (measured solid)
- ❖ 4 tbsp tomato paste
- ❖ 1 tsp ground ginger
- ❖ 1 1/2 tsp garam masala
- ❖ 1/2 tsp medium chilli powder
- ❖ 1 1/3 tsp cumin (or 3/4 tsp ground cumin)
- ❖ 1 tsp turmeric
- ❖ a pinch of Cayenne pepper
- ❖ 1/2 tsp salt
- ❖ 1 tsp minced garlic (optional)
- ❖ 1/2 tbsp fresh herbs (coriander, parsley or mint - to use as a topping)

INSTRUCTIONS

1. Melt the coconut oil in a pot over medium heat, when it's warm add the finely chopped onion (and garlic, if you are using it) and cook, stirring frequently, for a couple of minutes.
2. Add the spices and the tomato paste: stir for approx. 1 minute until fragrant.
3. Reduce the heat and add in the same pot the coconut milk. Mix well and cook for approx. 10 minutes until you get a creamy sauce.
4. Add the cauliflower and cook for approx. 10 minutes or until tender. Add the olive oil and mix well.
5. Taste and adjust the amount of spices if needed.
6. Serve warm with fresh herbs on top.

296. Crispy Greek-style pie

Prep Time: 40 minutes | Servings: 02
Per Servings: Kcal: 501, Protein: 26g, Fat: 27g, Net Carb: 8g

INGREDIENTS

- ❖ 200g (6 cup) bag spinach leaves
- ❖ 175g (6 cup) jar sundried tomato in oil
- ❖ 100g (1/2 cup) feta cheese, crumbled
- ❖ 2 eggs
- ❖ 125g (4/3 cup) filo pastry

INSTRUCTIONS

1. Put the spinach into a large pan. Pour over a couple tbsp water, then cook until just wilted. Tip into a sieve, leave to cool a little, then squeeze out any excess water and roughly chop. Roughly chop the tomatoes and put into a bowl along with the spinach, feta and eggs. Mix well.
2. Carefully unroll the filo pastry. Cover with some damp sheets of kitchen paper to stop it drying out. Take a sheet of pastry and brush liberally with some of the sundried tomato oil. Drape oil-side down in a 22cm loosebottomed cake tin so that some of the pastry hangs over the side. Brush oil on another piece of pastry and place in the tin, just a little further round. Keep placing the pastry pieces in the tin until you have roughly three layers, then spoon over the filling. Pull the sides into the middle, scrunch up and make sure the filling is covered. Brush with a little more oil.
3. Heat oven to 180C/fan 160C/gas 4. Cook the pie for 30 mins until the pastry is crisp and golden brown. Remove from the cake tin, slice into wedges and serve with salad.

Snack and Desserts Recipes

297. Fat Bombs

Prep Time: 15 minutes | Servings: 8 bombs
Per Bombs: Kcal: 126, Protein: 0g, Fat: 11g, Net Carb: 0g

INGREDIENTS

- ❖ ¼ cup (25g) cocoa butter
- ❖ ¼ cup (35g) coconut oil
- ❖ 10 drops vanilla stevia drops

INSTRUCTIONS

1. Melt together cocoa butter and coconut oil over low heat or in double boiler.
2. Remove from heat and stir in vanilla flavored stevia drops.
3. Pour into molds.
4. Chill until hardened.

5. Remove from molds and keep stored in the refrigerator.

298. Chocolate Chip Cookies

Prep Time: 15 minutes | **Servings:** 30 cookies
Per Cookies: Kcal: 125, Protein: 2g, Fat: 7g, Net Carb: 4g

INGREDIENTS

- ❖ 150g (3/4 cup) salted butter, softened
- ❖ 80g (1/2 cup) light brown muscovado sugar
- ❖ 80g (1/2 cup) granulated sugar
- ❖ 2 tsp vanilla extract
- ❖ 1 large egg
- ❖ 225g (1 cup) plain flour
- ❖ ½ tsp bicarbonate of soda
- ❖ ¼ tsp salt
- ❖ 200g (7 oz) plain chocolate chips or chunks

INSTRUCTIONS

1. Heat the oven to 190C/fan170C/gas 5 and line two baking sheets with non-stick baking paper.
2. Put 150g softened salted butter, 80g light brown muscovado sugar and 80g granulated sugar into a bowl and beat until creamy.
3. Beat in 2 tsp vanilla extract and 1 large egg.
4. Sift 225g plain flour, ½ tsp bicarbonate of soda and ¼ tsp salt into the bowl and mix it in with a wooden spoon.
5. Add 200g plain chocolate chips or chunks and stir well.
6. Use a teaspoon to make small scoops of the mixture, spacing them well apart on the baking trays. This mixture should make about 30 cookies.
7. Bake for 8–10 mins until they are light brown on the edges and still slightly soft in the centre if you press them.
8. Leave on the tray for a couple of mins to set and then lift onto a cooling rack.

299. Keto Cups

Prep Time: 30 minutes | **Servings:** 18 cups
Per Cups: Kcal: 120, Protein: 2g, Fat: 10g, Net Carb: 3g

INGREDIENTS

- ❖ 2 cups keto chocolate chips
- ❖ 1/4 tsp coconut oil
- ❖ 1/2 cup/115g coconut butter softened

INSTRUCTIONS

1. Line a 18-count mini muffin tin with mini muffin liners and set aside.
2. In a microwave safe bowl or stove top, melt your coconut oil with chocolate chips.
3. Moving quickly, coat the bottom and sides of the muffin liners with melted chocolate. Ensure a little is leftover to top with later. Place the chocolate coated muffin tins in the freezer to firm up.
4. Once firm, drizzle the coconut butter amongst the cups. Top with the remaining chocolate and freeze until firm.

300. Chip Cookie

Prep Time: 20 minutes | **Servings:** 18 Cookies
Per Cookies: Kcal: 137, Protein: 2g, Fat: 11g, Net Carb: 0.5g

INGREDIENTS

- ❖ 1/2 cup (110g) butter softened
- ❖ 1/3 cup (40g) Swerve confectioners' sugar (Erythritol sweetener)
- ❖ 1 teaspoon pure vanilla extract
- ❖ 1/2 teaspoon kosher salt
- ❖ 2 cup (225g) almond flour
- ❖ 9 ounces idark chocolate chips
- ❖ 8 ounces sugar-free chocolate chips

INSTRUCTIONS

1. In a large bowl beat butter until light and fluffy, using a hand mixer. Mix in sugar, salt, and vanilla and mix until combined.
2. Add in almond flour a little at a time and mix until dough consistency forms. Pour in dark chocolate chips and mix. Cover with plastic wrap and place in the refrigerator for 10-15 minutes.
3. Remove dough from fridge and use a cookie scoop or measuring spoon to form 1-inch balls (about 1 heaping tablespoon). Place on

a rimmed baking sheet lined with parchment paper.

4. In a microwave-safe dish melt, sugar-free chocolate chips in 30-second increments, stirring between each round of heating until smooth.

5. Dip each chilled fat bomb in melted chocolate and then put back onto the lined baking sheet. Place in freezer for 5 minutes, or until chocolate has hardened.

301. Keto Brownie Cookies

Prep Time: 20 minutes | **Servings:** 18 Cookies
Per Cookies: Kcal: 57, Protein: 12g, Fat: 19g, Net Carb: 1g

INGREDIENTS

- ❖ 4 oz cream cheese, room temperature
- ❖ 1/3 cup (40g) Swerve confectioners sweetener
- ❖ 1 egg, beaten
- ❖ 1 teaspoon baking powder
- ❖ 6 tablespoons cocoa powder
- ❖ 1/3 cup (55g) ChocZero or Lilys low carb chocolate chips
- ❖ ¼ teaspoon SweetLeaf vanilla liquid stevia

INSTRUCTIONS

1. Preheat oven to 350 degrees F. Line a cookie sheet with parchment paper and set aside.

2. Using a hand mixer, cream the Swerve sweetener and cream cheese. When nice and creamy add in the baking powder, stevia, cocoa powder and egg.

3. Mix well until a dough forms. Add the chocolate chips and mix with a spoon to incorporate.

4. Spoon out the cookies on the cookie sheet. The dough is very sticky. Flatten the cookie dough with your fingers. Or take a piece of wax paper and spray it generously with cooking spray. Then place it on the cookies and flatten them with your hand. That way you won't get your hands messy.

5. Bake for 8-10 minutes. You want the cookies to be firm to the touch but not too firm.

6. Take out of the oven and let cool completely before eating. Eat immediately or store in the refrigerator or freezer.

7. For the chocolate chips I used low carb ChocZero or Lily's dark chocolate stevia sweetened mini chips.

302. Butter Fat Bombs

Prep Time: 20 minutes | **Servings:** 12 Boms
Per Bombs: Kcal: 167, Protein: 1g, Fat: 19g, Net Carb: 1g

INGREDIENTS

- ❖ 2 cups/460g heavy whipping cream/double cream (very cold)
- ❖ 1 teaspoon vanilla
- ❖ 2 to 3 tablespoons sweetener {to taste}
- ❖ 3 tablespoons peanut butter

INSTRUCTIONS

1. Place the cold whipping cream in a medium mixing bowl mixing at medium speed.

2. Add the vanilla. At the soft peak stage add the sugar substitute followed by the peanut butter.

3. Whip until combined.

4. Place 12 cupcake liners in a muffin tin. Set aside.

5. Using a plastic baggie or icing bag, pipe peanut butter mixture into liners.

6. Place into freezer for 2 hours or until frozen. Then place in a sealed container in the freezer for storage.

303. No Bake Cookies

Prep Time: 30 minutes | **Servings:** 48 Cookies
Per Cookies: Kcal: 71, Protein: 1g, Fat: 9g, Net Carb: 0.2g

INGREDIENTS

- ❖ 3/4 cup (240ml) coconut oil
- ❖ 3/4 cup (85g) creamy low carb peanut butter or almond butter
- ❖ 1/4 cup (25g) cocoa powder
- ❖ 1 cup (125g) swerve sweetener (brown sugar or granular)
- ❖ 1 teaspoon vanilla extract (optional)

- ❖ 1 1/2 cup (105g) UNSWEETENED coconut flakes
- ❖ 2 tablespoons hulled hemp seeds, also called hemp hearts (you can use an extra 2 tablespoons of coconut flakes if you don't have this. I like the mixed texture and it adds a bit of fiber)
- ❖ sea salt for topping (optional)

INSTRUCTIONS

1. In a medium size sauce pan combine the coconut oil and the peanut butter over medium low heat.
2. As the mixture begins to melt stir until well combined.
3. Stir in the cocoa powder, vanilla (if using) and the .
4. Increase heat to medium or just over medium and slowly bring the mixture to a simmer.
5. When the mixture is simmering and the sweetener has completely melted (your fudge mixture should be smooth with no visible granulars) remove from heat and stir in the coconut flakes and the hemp seeds.
6. Set aside and allow mixture to cool slightly.
7. Carefully spoon into silicone mini muffin tins until 3/4 full.
8. Sprinkle with sea salt if desired.
9. Freeze for 15 minutes until set. Remove from tins and store in an air tight container in the freezer.

304. Cheesecake Bites

Prep Time: 30 minutes | Servings: 20 Bites
Per Bites: Kcal: 36, Protein: 1g, Fat: 2g, Net Carb: 0.2g

INGREDIENTS

- ❖ 3.4 ounces package low-carb/sugar-free instant chocolate pudding
- ❖ 8 ounces cream cheese (room temperature)
- ❖ 1 teaspoon vanilla extract
- ❖ 1/4 teaspoon salt
- ❖ 1/3 cup (35g) Powdered Erythritol Sweetener (or Powdered Swerve Sweetener)
- ❖ 1/3 cup (35g) unsweetened cocoa powder

INSTRUCTIONS

1. In a medium bowl, mix the chocolate pudding, cream cheese, vanilla, salt, powdered sugar.
2. Chill the mixture for 30 minutes.
3. Add cocoa powder to a small bowl.
4. Use a 1 tablespoon cookie scoop to form the dough into balls then dip in a small bowl of cocoa powder until coated.
5. Chill for 30 minutes and enjoy!

305. Chocolate Fat Bombs

Prep Time: 20 minutes | Servings: 10 Boms
Per Boms: Kcal: 46, Protein: 1g, Fat: 1g, Net Carb: 0.4g

INGREDIENTS

- ❖ 1/2 cup (120ml) coconut oil
- ❖ 1/2 cup (60g) swerve sweetener (granular and brown sugar work)
- ❖ 1/2 cup (125g) low carb peanut butter
- ❖ 3/4 cup (110g) Lilly's Dark Chocolate Chips

INSTRUCTIONS

1. Heat a medium size sauce pan to medium low heat.
2. Add the coconut oil first and wait until it has completely melted.
3. Then add the sugar substitute, peanut butter and chocolate chips.
4. Stir the mixture continuously until it has completely melted.
5. Remove from heat and allow mixture to cool 5-10 minutes.
6. Carefully spoon into a silicone mini muffin tin until 3/4 full. (This makes 34 for me)
7. Sprinkle with sea salt if desired.
8. Freeze until firm.

306. Smores Recipe

Prep Time: 20 minutes | Servings: 4
Per Servings: Kcal: 150, Protein: 6g, Fat: 15g, Net Carb: 0.6g

INGREDIENTS

- ❖ 12 Keto Graham Crackers
- ❖ 6 squares Lindt 90% Dark Chocolate
- ❖ 6 Keto Marshmallows

INSTRUCTIONS

1. Place 6 crackers onto a cookie sheet lined with parchment paper, top each with the square of chocolate.
2. Grill/Broil for 3-5 minutes until the chocolate has melted slightly.
3. Top each with a marshmallow, followed by another graham cracker.
4. Enjoy immediately.

307. Strawberry Cheesecake

Prep Time: 25 minutes | **Servings:** 2
Per Servings: Kcal: 201, Protein: 6g, Fat: 30g, Net Carb: 0.7g

INGREDIENTS

- ❖ 8 oz. cream cheese, room temperature
- ❖ ⅓ cup (35g) fresh or frozen strawberries
- ❖ 4 tbsp unsalted butter
- ❖ 1 scoop Vanilla MCT Powder
- ❖ 1 tbsp monk fruit (or another low carb sweetener)
- ❖ Splash of vanilla extract or the paste of 1/2

INSTRUCTIONS

1. Puree the strawberries in a small blender or using a hand mixer.
2. Add a small splash of vanilla and mix to incorporate.
3. Prepare a muffin tray with muffin liners.
4. Melt the cream cheese and butter together.
5. In a medium-sized mixing bowl, combine the dairy mixture and the strawberry mixture, and mix well.
6. Pour evenly in muffin tins or silicone mold and place in the freezer to chill for no less than 40 minutes.

308. Chocolate Chip

Prep Time: 20 minutes | **Servings:** 10 Chips

Per Chips: Kcal: 286, Protein: 1g, Fat: 1g, Net Carb: 4g

INGREDIENTS

Crust
- ❖ 8 tablespoons butter (1 stick)
- ❖ 1 ¼ cup/140g almond flour
- ❖ 2 tablespoons swerve

Cheesecake Filling:
- ❖ 2 8oz packages cream cheese
- ❖ 1 egg
- ❖ 1 tablespoon vanilla
- ❖ ½ cup/60g powdered swerve (confectioners' sugar)
- ❖ 1 cup/150g chocolate chip (lily's sugar-free)

INSTRUCTIONS

1. Preheat oven to 350°
2. Line a 9x9 baking pan with parchment paper or aluminum foil, lightly spray with cooking spray and set aside.
3. Melt butter
4. Combine butter, almond flour and swerve. Mix well.
5. Pat crust into pan and bake for 6 minutes
6. Cheesecake Filling
7. Combine cream cheese, egg, vanilla, and powdered swerve in a bowl and beat with an electric mixer until well combined
8. Fold in chocolate chips
9. Evenly press the cheesecake filling into the pan and bake 30 minutes until a toothpick placed in the center comes out clean.

309. Peanut Butter Chocolate Bars

Prep Time: 30 minutes | **Servings:** 8 Bars
Per Bars: Kcal: 246, Protein: 7g, Fat: 23g, Net Carb: 6g

INGREDIENTS

For the Bars
- ❖ 3/4 cup (84 g) Superfine Almond Flour
- ❖ 2 oz (56.7 g) Butter
- ❖ 1/4 cup (45.5 g) Swerve, Icing sugar style
- ❖ 1/2 cup (129 g) Creamy Peanut Butter
- ❖ 1 tsp Vanilla extract

For the Topping
- 1/2 cup (90 g) Sugar-Free Chocolate Chips

INSTRUCTIONS:

1. Mix all the ingredients for the bars together and spread into a small 6-inch pan
2. Melt the chocolate chips in a microwave oven for 30 seconds and stir.
3. Add another 10 seconds if needed to melt fully.
4. Spread the topping on top of the bars.
5. Refrigerate for at least an hour or two until the bars thicken up. These bars definitely improve with keeping so don't be in a huge rush to eat them.

310. Keto Chocolate Mousse

Prep Time: 12 minutes | Servings: 2
Per Servings: Kcal: 373, Protein: 5g, Fat: 37g, Net Carb: 6g

INGREDIENTS

- 3 ounces cream cheese, softened
- ½ cup (115g) heavy cream/double cream
- 1 teaspoon vanilla extract
- ¼ cup (6g) powdered zero-calorie sweetener
- 2 tablespoons cocoa powder
- 1 pinch salt

INSTRUCTIONS

1. Place cream cheese in a large bowl and beat using an electric mixer until light and fluffy. Turn mixer to low speed and slowly add heavy cream and vanilla extract. Add sweetener, cocoa powder and salt, mixing until well incorporated. Turn mixer to high, and mix until light and fluffy, 1 to 2 minutes more. Serve immediately, or refrigerate for later.

311. Chocolate Crunch Bars

Prep Time: 30 minutes | Servings: 20 Bars
Per Bars: Kcal: 156, Protein: 6g, Fat: 12g, Net Carb: 4g

INGREDIENTS

- 1 1/2 cups (225g) chocolate chips of choice I used stevia sweetened keto friendly chocolate chips
- 1 cup (112g) almond butter Can sub for any nut or seed butter of choice
- 1/2 cup (12g) sticky sweetener of choice
- 1/4 cup (60ml) coconut oil
- 3 cups (450g) nuts and seeds of choice almonds, cashews, pepitas etc

INSTRUCTIONS

1. Line an 8 x 8-inch baking dish with parchment paper and set aside.
2. In a microwave-safe bowl or stovetop, combine your chocolate chips of choice, almond butter, sticky sweetener and coconut oil and melt until combined.
3. Add your nuts/seeds of choice and mix until fully combined. Pour the keto crunch bar mixture into the lined baking dish and spread out using a spatula. Refrigerate or freeze until firm.

312. Keto Lemon Bars

Prep Time: 50 minutes | Servings: 08 Bars
Per Bars: Kcal: 272, Protein: 8g, Fat: 26g, Net Carb: 4g

INGREDIENTS

- 1/2 cup (120g) butter, melted
- 1 3/4 cups (200g) almond flour
- 1 cup (100g) powdered erythritol
- 3 medium lemons
- 3 large eggs

INSTRUCTIONS

1. Mix butter, 1 cup almond flour, 1/4 cup erythritol, and a pinch of salt. Press evenly into an 8x8" parchment paper-lined baking dish. Bake for 20 minutes at 350 degrees F. Then, let cool for 10 minutes.
2. Into a bowl, zest one of the lemons, then juice all 3 lemons, add the eggs, 3/4 cup erythritol, 3/4 cup almond flour & pinch of salt. Combine to make filling.
3. Pour the filling onto the crust & bake for 25 minutes.

4. Serve with lemon slices and a sprinkle of erythritol.

313. Keto Chocolate

Prep Time: 10 minutes | Servings: 12 chocolates
Per Chocolate: Kcal: 81, Protein: 0.5g, Fat: 9g, Net Carb: 1g

INGREDIENTS

- ❖ 3.5 oz/100g cacao butter
- ❖ 6 tbsp (48g) cocoa powder unsweetened
- ❖ 4 tbsp (32g) powdered erythritol (So nourished)

INSTRUCTIONS

1. Melt the cacao butter in a pan, stirring continuously.
2. Add the cocoa powder and powdered erythritol and stir until combined.
3. Add any optional extra (1 tsp orange zest/pinch cinnamon/pinch of sea salt/pinch of chili/1/3 cup (50g) low carb granola/handful of nuts and seeds and stir
4. Fill into a silicone chocolate mould to make chocolate bars. Or pour onto parchment paper to make chocolate bark/clusters.
5. Freeze 5 minutes until set.

314. Chocolate Fat Bombs

Prep Time: 10 minutes | Servings: 16 bomns
Per Bombs: Kcal: 90, Protein: 3g, Fat: 8g, Net Carb: 1g

INGREDIENTS

- ❖ 120g (1 cup) Almond Butter (100% nuts) - this can be swapped for any other nut butter
- ❖ 60g (1/4 cup) Coconut Oil or Unsalted Butter
- ❖ 40ml Coconut Milk or Double Cream
- ❖ 20g (1/4 cup) Cocoa Powder
- ❖ 20g (1/3 cup) Truvia / Pure Via Sweetener
- ❖ 1/2 tsp Vanilla Extract

INSTRUCTIONS

1. Melt the almond butter and coconut oil either in the microwave or in a non-stick saucepan.

2. Transfer these to a mixing bowl, add all of the remaining ingredients and mix. The texture will change to a thick mousse.
3. Line a small tray with greaseproof paper and spread the mix evenly, or use silicone moulds like those shown in the picture.
4. Store these in the freezer - they'll take about an hour to set. They'll melt if left outside of the freezer.

315. Chocolate Fat Bombs

Prep Time: 10 minutes | Servings: 1
Per Serving: Kcal: 116, Protein: 2g, Fat: 11g, Net Carb: 3g

INGREDIENTS

- ❖ 1/2 Tbsp melted organic coconut oil
- ❖ 1/2 Tbsp organic cacao powder
- ❖ 1/2 Tbsp almond butter
- ❖ 1–3 drops liquid stevia,

INSTRUCTIONS

1. Melt the coconut oil, stir in the cacao and almond butter, and eat right away.

316. Blueberry & pecan cookies

Prep Time: 30 minutes | Servings: 12 chocolates
Per Chocolate: Kcal: 270, Protein: 4g, Fat: 14g, Net Carb: 10g

INGREDIENTS

- ❖ 175g (1 cup) plain flour, plus extra for dusting
- ❖ ½ tsp baking powder
- ❖ 85g (1 cup) porridge oat
- ❖ 175g (4/5 cup) golden caster sugar
- ❖ 1 tsp ground cinnamon
- ❖ 140g (1/2 cup) butter, chopped
- ❖ 70g (1 cup) pack dried blueberry (or use raisins or dried cranberries)
- ❖ 50g (1/2 cup) pecan, roughly broken
- ❖ 1 egg, beaten

INSTRUCTIONS

1. Tip the flour, baking powder, oats, sugar and cinnamon into a bowl, then mix well with your hands. Add the butter, then rub it into the mixture until it has disappeared.

2. Stir in the blueberries and pecans, add the egg, then mix well with a cutlery knife or wooden spoon until it all comes together in a big ball. Lightly flour the work surface, then roll the dough into a fat sausage about 6cm across. Wrap in cling film, then chill in the fridge until solid.

3. To bake, heat oven to 180C/fan 160C/ gas 4. Unwrap the cookie log, thickly slice into discs, then arrange on baking sheets. Bake for 15 mins (or a few mins more if from frozen) until golden, leave on the trays to harden, then cool completely on a wire rack before tucking in.

Keto Soup Recipes

317. Broccoli & Pea Soup

Prep Time: 30 minutes | **Servings:** 2
Per Serving: Kcal: 280, Protein: 20g, Fat: 16g, Net Carb: 8g

INGREDIENTS

- ❖ 1 tbsp rapeseed oil
- ❖ 1 onion, finely chopped
- ❖ 1 large garlic clove, crushed
- ❖ 400g (14 oz.) broccoli, chopped into small florets
- ❖ 300g (10 oz.) frozen peas
- ❖ 200g (3/2 cup) chard, chopped
- ❖ 1l low-salt veg stock
- ❖ ½ small bunch of basil, chopped
- ❖ small bunch of dill, chopped
- ❖ 1 lemon, zested and juiced
- ❖ 2 tbsp pumpkin seeds, toasted

INSTRUCTIONS

1. Heat the oil in a large saucepan. Add the onion and fry for 8 mins until soft and translucent. Add the garlic and cook for 1 min more. Tip in the broccoli, peas and chard, then pour over the stock and bring the mixture to the boil. Reduce the heat to a simmer, cover and cook for 25 mins.

2. Stir through the herbs, lemon zest and juice, then blitz the soup with a stick blender until completely smooth. Ladle into bowls and serve with the toasted pumpkin seeds scattered over the top.

318. Green Vegetable Soup

Prep Time: 30 minutes | **Servings:** 4
Per Serving: Kcal: 150, Protein: 10g, Fat: 15g, Net Carb: 8g

INGREDIENTS

- ❖ 1 bunch spring onions, chopped
- ❖ 1large potato, peeled and chopped
- ❖ 1 garlic clove, crushed
- ❖ 1l vegetable stock
- ❖ 250g (8.4 oz.) frozen peas
- ❖ 100g (3.4 oz.) fresh spinach
- ❖ 300ml natural yogurt
- ❖ few mint leaves, basil leaves, cress or a mixture, to serve

INSTRUCTIONS

1. Put the spring onions, potato and garlic into a large pan. Pour over the vegetable stock and bring to the boil.

2. Reduce the heat and simmer for 15 mins with a lid on or until the potato is soft enough to mash with the back of a spoon.

3. Add the peas and bring back up to a simmer. Scoop out around 4 tbsp of the peas and set aside for the garnish.

4. Stir the spinach and yogurt into the pan, then carefully pour the whole mixture into a blender or use a stick blender to blitz it until it's very smooth. Season to taste with black pepper.

5. Ladle into bowls, then add some of the reserved cooked peas and scatter over your favourite soft herbs or cress. Serve with crusty bread, if you like.

319. Keto Chicken Soup

Prep Time: 60 minutes | **Servings:** 04
Per Serving: Kcal: 272, Protein: 31g, Fat: 12g, Net Carb: 9g

INGREDIENTS

- ❖ 2 tbsp. vegetable oil
- ❖ 1 medium onion, chopped

- ❖ 5 cloves garlic, smashed
- ❖ 2"-piece fresh ginger, sliced
- ❖ 1 small cauliflower, cut into florets
- ❖ 3/4 tsp. crushed red pepper flakes
- ❖ 1 medium carrot, peeled and thinly sliced on a bias
- ❖ 6 cup (570g) low-sodium chicken broth
- ❖ 1 stalk celery, thinly sliced
- ❖ 2 boneless skinless chicken breasts
- ❖ Freshly chopped parsley, for garnish

INSTRUCTIONS

1. In a large pot over medium heat, heat oil. Add onion, garlic and ginger. Cook until beginning to brown.
2. Meanwhile, pulse cauliflower in a food processor until broken down into rice-sized granules. Add cauliflower to pot with onion mixture and cook over medium high heat until beginning to brown, about 8 minutes.
3. Add pepper flakes, carrots, celery and chicken broth and bring to a simmer. Add chicken breasts and let cook gently until they reach an internal temperature of 165°, about 15 minutes. Remove from pan, let cool until cool enough to handle, and shred. Meanwhile, continue simmering until vegetables are tender, 3 to 5 minutes more.
4. Remove ginger from pot, and add shredded chicken back to soup. Season to taste with salt and pepper, then garnish with parsley before serving.

320. Keto Zuppa Toscana

Prep Time: 40 minutes | Servings: 04
Per Serving: Kcal: 439, Protein: 18g, Fat: 37g, Net Carb: 5g

INGREDIENTS

- ❖ 1 lb mild Italian Sausage
- ❖ 4 slices thick-cut bacon
- ❖ 32 oz Beef bone broth (or beef broth)
- ❖ 1 small onion, diced
- ❖ 3 cloves fresh garlic, minced
- ❖ 1 head fresh cauliflower, diced
- ❖ ½ cup/115g heavy whipping cream/double cream

- ❖ 2 cups (60g) fresh spinach (5 oz package), or kale

INSTRUCTIONS

1. Using a large soup pot, brown your sausage and bacon together. Cut your bacon into bite sized pieces to make it easier to cook.
2. Once your meat is cooked, add in beef bone broth, onions, garlic, and cauliflower. Cover and cook on medium heat for about 15 minutes, until the cauliflower is tender.
3. Once the cauliflower is softened, add in heavy cream and spinach (or kale). Cook for about 5 minutes, until spinach (or kale) is soft.
4. Serve with a spinkle of parmesan cheese and a pinch of salt, pepper, and/or crushed red pepper flakes. ENJOY!

321. Vegetable Soup Recipe

Prep Time: 35 minutes | Servings: 12
Per Serving: Kcal: 80, Protein: 3g, Fat: 2g, Net Carb: 6g

INGREDIENTS

- ❖ 2 tbsp Olive oil
- ❖ 1 large Onion (diced)
- ❖ 2 large Bell peppers (diced, the same size as onions)
- ❖ 4 cloves Garlic (minced)
- ❖ 1 medium head Cauliflower (cut into 1-inch florets)
- ❖ 2 cups (300g) green beans (trimmed, cut into 1-inch pieces)
- ❖ 2 14.5-oz cans Diced tomatoes
- ❖ 8 cups (770g) Chicken broth (or vegetable broth for vegetarian/vegan)
- ❖ 1 tbsp Italian seasoning
- ❖ 2 Dried Bay leaves (optional)
- ❖ Sea salt (optional, to taste)
- ❖ Black pepper (optional, to taste)

INSTRUCTIONS

1. Heat olive oil in a pot or dutch oven over medium heat.
2. Add the onions and bell peppers. Saute for 7 to 10 minutes, until onions are translucent and browned.

3. Add the minced garlic. Saute for about a minute, until fragrant.
4. Add the cauliflower, green beans, diced tomatoes, broth, and Italian seasoning. Adjust sea salt and black pepper to taste. Add the bay leaves, if using.
5. Bring the soup to a boil. Cover, reduce heat to medium low, and cook for about 10 to 20 minutes, until veggies are soft.

322. Broccoli Cheddar Soup

Prep Time: 25 minutes | **Servings:** 4
Per Serving: Kcal: 282, Protein: 12g, Fat: 24g, Net Carb: 1g

INGREDIENTS

- ❖ 2 tablespoons Butter
- ❖ 1/ 8 Cup (20g) White Onion
- ❖ 1/2 teaspoon Garlic, finely minced
- ❖ 2 Cups (200g) Chicken Broth
- ❖ Salt and Pepper, to taste
- ❖ 1 Cup (70g) Broccoli, chopped into bite size pieces
- ❖ 1 Tablespoon Cream Cheese
- ❖ 1/4 Cup (58g) Heavy Whipping Cream/double cream
- ❖ 1 Cup (112g) Cheddar Cheese; shredded

INSTRUCTIONS

1. In large pot, saute onion and garlic with butter over medium heat until onions are softened and translucent.
2. Add broth and broccoli to pot. Cook broccoli until tender. Add salt, pepper and desired seasoning.
3. Place cream cheese in small bowl and heat in microwave for ~30 seconds until soft and easily stirred.
4. Stir heavy whipping cream and cream cheese into soup; bring to a boil.
5. Turn off heat and quickly stir in cheddar cheese.
6. Stir in xanthan gum, if desired. Allow to thicken.

323. Butter Mushroom Soup

Prep Time: 25 minutes | **Servings:** 6

Per Serving: Kcal: 198, Protein: 5g, Fat: 18g, Net Carb: 4g

INGREDIENTS

- ❖ 6 tablespoon (113.5g) butters
- ❖ 2 tablespoon fresh sage chopped
- ❖ 1 lb mushrooms sliced
- ❖ 4 cups (390g) vegetable or chicken broth
- ❖ Salt and pepper to taste
- ❖ ½ cup (115g) heavy cream/double cream

INSTRUCTIONS

1. In a large pot, heat butter over medium heat until it begins to brown and turns fragrant, 3 to 4 minutes. Add sage and cook one minute more.
2. Add mushrooms and stir to coat, then saute until mushrooms are tender and lightly browned, 4 to 5 minutes.
3. Stir in stock and bring to a simmer. Cook 4 to 5 minutes more.
4. Transfer to food processor or blender (in batches, if your processor is not large enough). Blend until smooth.
5. Return to pot and stir in cream. Serve immediately.

324. Asparagus Soup

Prep Time: 40 minutes | **Servings:** 4
Per Serving: Kcal: 210, Protein: 8g, Fat: 16g, Net Carb: 4g

INGREDIENTS

- ❖ 2 tbsp. butter
- ❖ 1 clove garlic, minced
- ❖ 2 lb. asparagus, ends trimmed, cut into 1" pieces
- ❖ Kosher salt
- ❖ Freshly ground black pepper
- ❖ 2 cup (200g) low-sodium chicken broth
- ❖ 1/2 cup (115g) heavy cream or double cream, plus more for garnish
- ❖ Freshly chopped chives, for garnish
- ❖ Freshly chopped dill, for garnish

INSTRUCTIONS

1. In a heavy pot over medium heat, melt butter. Add garlic and cook until fragrant, 1

minute. Add asparagus, season with salt and pepper, and cook until golden, 5 minutes. Add broth and simmer, covered, until asparagus is very tender but still green, 10 to 15 minutes.

2. Using an immersion or regular blender, puree soup. If using a regular blender, be sure to stop and remove lid a few times to avoid overheating the soup. Return to pot, stir in cream, then warm over low heat. Season with salt and pepper to taste.
3. Garnish with more cream and herbs.

325. Chicken Coconut Soup

Prep Time: 40 minutes | Servings: 4
Per Serving: Kcal: 436, Protein: 32g, Fat: 33g, Net Carb: 8g

INGREDIENTS

- ❖ 1 tbsp. extra-virgin olive oil
- ❖ 1 tbsp. freshly minced ginger
- ❖ 4 oz. shiitake mushrooms, chopped
- ❖ 6 cup (580g) low-sodium chicken broth
- ❖ 1 (14-oz.) can coconut milk
- ❖ 1 tbsp. fish sauce
- ❖ 1 lb. boneless skinless chicken thighs, cut into 1" pieces
- ❖ Juice of 1 lime
- ❖ Cilantro leaves, for garnish

INSTRUCTIONS

1. In a large pot over medium heat, heat oil. Add ginger and cook until fragrant, 1 minute, then add mushrooms and cook until soft, about 6 minutes.
2. Add broth, coconut milk, and fish sauce and bring to a boil. Add chicken, reduce heat, and simmer until chicken is no longer pink, about 15 minutes. Turn off heat and stir in lime juice.
3. Garnish with cilantro and chili oil (if using) before serving.

326. Broccoli And Stilton Soup

Prep Time: 30 minutes | Servings: 2
Per Serving: Kcal: 375, Protein: 32g, Fat: 28g, Net Carb: 2g

INGREDIENTS

- ❖ 1 onion, finely chopped
- ❖ 1 celery stick, sliced
- ❖ 1 leek, sliced
- ❖ 1 medium potato, diced
- ❖ 750ml low salt or homemade chicken or vegetable stock
- ❖ 1 head broccoli, roughly chopped
- ❖ 140g (3/2 cup) stilton, or other blue cheese, crumbled

INSTRUCTIONS

1. Put all the ingredients into the soup maker, except the stilton, and press the 'smooth soup' function. Make sure you don't fill the soup maker above the max fill line.
2. Once the cycle is complete, season, and stir in most of the stilton. Blend briefly again until the cheese has melted into the soup. Season with more black pepper and top with the reserved cheese to serve.

327. Keto Turkey Soup

Prep Time: 20 minutes | Servings: 4
Per Serving: Kcal: 290, Protein: 26g, Fat: 17g, Net Carb: 3g

INGREDIENTS

- ❖ 1 tablespoon butter
- ❖ 1 tablespoon olive oil
- ❖ ½ cup (25g) onion chopped
- ❖ ½ cup (4 oz.) celery chopped
- ❖ ¼ cup (30 g) carrot chopped
- ❖ 8 oz cauliflower rice
- ❖ 1 quart chicken or turkey stock
- ❖ 2 cups (260g) dark cooked turkey meat shredded
- ❖ 1 tablespoon salt
- ❖ 1 teaspoon pepper
- ❖ 1 teaspoon garlic powder
- ❖ 1 teaspoon dried dill
- ❖ ½ cup (120 ml) heavy cream/double cream
- ❖ ½ cup (70g) crumbled bacon

INSTRUCTIONS

1. Heat the oil in a large saucepan

over a medium heat, tip in the celery, garlic and potatoes and coat in the oil. Add a splash of water and a big pinch of salt and cook, stirring regularly for 15 mins, adding a little more water if the veg begins to stick.

2. Pour in the vegetable stock and bring to the boil, then turn the heat down and simmer for 20 mins further, until the potatoes are falling apart and the celery is soft. Use a stick blender to purée the soup, then pour in the milk and blitz again. Season to taste. Serve with crusty bread.

328. Chilled green soup

Prep Time: 25 minutes | Servings: 4
Per Serving: Kcal: 400, Protein: 11g, Fat: 34g, Net Carb: 2g

INGREDIENTS

- ❖ 70g (1/2 cup) vegetarian feta, crumbled
- ❖ 3 tbsp olive oil
- ❖ 1 tsp coriander seeds, crushed
- ❖ 1 large red chilli, deseeded and finely chopped
- ❖ 1 lemon, zested and juiced
- ❖ 200g (5 cup) baby spinach
- ❖ 2 large ripe avocados, stoned and cubed
- ❖ 1 large cucumber, chopped
- ❖ 1 small garlic clove, crushed
- ❖ 250g (1 cup) natural yogurt
- ❖ small bunch basil
- ❖ 2 tbsp toasted mixed seeds, to serve

INSTRUCTIONS

1. Put the feta in a bowl and pour over the olive oil, coriander seeds, chilli and lemon zest. Set aside.
2. Tip the remaining ingredients (except the seeds) into a food processor and blitz until smooth. Season. Add 50-100ml cold water and blitz again to loosen. Chill for up to 1 hr.
3. Pour into four bowls and top with the feta, marinating liquid and seeds.

329. Vegetable Cabbage Soup

Prep Time: 40 minutes | Servings: 4

Per Serving: Kcal: 187, Protein: 11g, Fat: 8g, Net Carb: 7g

INGREDIENTS

- ❖ 2 tbsp. extra-virgin olive oil
- ❖ 1 large onion, chopped
- ❖ 2 carrots, chopped
- ❖ 2 stalks celery, minced
- ❖ 1/2 tsp. chili powder
- ❖ Kosher salt
- ❖ Freshly ground black pepper
- ❖ 1 (15-oz.) can white beans, drained and rinsed
- ❖ 2 cloves garlic, minced
- ❖ 1 tsp. thyme leaves
- ❖ 4 cup/400g low-sodium chicken broth
- ❖ 2 cup/500ml water
- ❖ 1/2 large head cabbage, chopped
- ❖ 1 (15-oz.) can chopped fire-roasted tomatoes
- ❖ Pinch red pepper flakes
- ❖ 2 tbsp. freshly chopped parsley, plus more for garnish

INSTRUCTIONS

1. In a large pot over medium heat, heat olive oil. Add onion, carrots, and celery, and season with salt, pepper, and chili powder. Cook, stirring often, until vegetables are soft, 5 to 6 minutes. Stir in beans, garlic, and thyme and cook until garlic is fragrant, about 30 seconds. Add broth and water, and bring to a simmer.
2. Stir in tomatoes and cabbage and simmer until cabbage is wilted, about 6 minutes.
3. Remove from heat and stir in red pepper flakes, and parsley. Season to taste with salt and pepper. Garnish with more parsley, if using.

330. Tomato Soup

Prep Time: 45 minutes | Servings: 4
Per Serving: Kcal: 95, Protein: 3g, Fat: 5g, Net Carb: 1g

INGREDIENTS

- ❖ 1 tbsp. extra-virgin olive oil, plus more for garnish
- ❖ 1 small yellow onion, chopped
- ❖ 2 garlic cloves, minced

- ❖ 1/2 tsp. crushed red pepper flakes
- ❖ 2 tbsp. tomato paste
- ❖ 1 tsp. fresh thyme leaves, plus more for garnish
- ❖ 2 (28-oz.) cans whole peeled tomatoes
- ❖ Kosher salt
- ❖ Freshly ground black pepper
- ❖ 2 cup (500 ml) water or vegetable stock

INSTRUCTIONS

1. In a large pot over medium heat, heat oil. Add onion and cook until soft, 6 minutes. Add garlic, red pepper flakes, and tomato paste and cook until garlic is fragrant and tomato paste has darkened, 2 to 3 minutes more.
2. Add thyme and both cans tomatoes, including the juice. Add water or vegetable stock and bring up to a simmer. Cook for 10 minutes.
3. Blend with immersion blender or transfer to a blender in batches and blend until smooth. Ladle into bowls and serve with a drizzle of olive oil and some fresh thyme leaves.

331. Keto Tomato Soup

Prep Time: 35 minutes | Servings: 4
Per Serving: Kcal: 140, Protein: 4g, Fat: 11g, Net Carb: 5g

INGREDIENTS

- ❖ 4 Medium Tomatoes (500g)
- ❖ 3 Tbsp/42g Olive Oil
- ❖ 5 Garlic Cloves (13g)
- ❖ 2 Cups (480mL) Chicken Broth
- ❖ 1 Tbsp/3g Herbs de Provence
- ❖ ½ Tsp Salt
- ❖ ¼ Tsp Black Pepper

INSTRUCTIONS

1. Preheat your oven to 400°F (204°C)
2. Place tomatoes and garlic cloves on a baking sheet. Drizzle with olive oil. Roast in the oven for 25 minutes...alternatively you can use canned tomatoes and pre-minced garlic as listed above.

3. If you used fresh tomatoes, discard the skins. Use a spatula to transfer the roasted tomatoes, garlic, and oil into a blender or food processor. Purée until smooth.
4. Pour the purée, broth, and seasonings into a small stockpot. Stir well. Bring to everything to a boil. Simmer for a bit longer if you prefer a thicker consistency. Serve hot!..

332. Cauliflower cheese soup

Prep Time: 35 minutes | Servings: 4
Per Serving: Kcal: 140, Protein: 4g, Fat: 11g, Net Carb: 5g

INGREDIENTS

- ❖ 2 tbsp rapeseed oil, plus 50ml extra
- ❖ 1 chopped onion
- ❖ 1 vegetable stock cube
- ❖ 1 large chopped head of cauliflower
- ❖ 400g (3/2 cup) can butter beans
- ❖ 400ml (2 cup) milk
- ❖ 800ml (3 cup) water
- ❖ grating fresh nutmeg
- ❖ 2 tsp Dijon mustard
- ❖ 50g extra mature cheddar
- ❖ 100ml (1/2 cup) double cream
- ❖ handful sage leaves
- ❖ chopped toasted hazelnuts

INSTRUCTIONS

1. Heat the rapeseed oil in a large pan and cook the onion until starting to caramelise. Add the vegetable stock cube, cauliflower and drained butter beans. Stir, then pour in the milk and water. Season and add a grating fresh nutmeg. Cover and simmer for 20 mins.
2. Blend the soup with a hand blender until smooth, adding more liquid if necessary. Add the Dijon mustard, extra mature cheddar and double cream. In another pan, sizzle a handful sage leaves in 50ml oil until crisp. Ladle the soup into bowls. Top with the sage, oil and some chopped toasted hazelnuts.

CONCLUSION

One of the primary keys to any successful diet or lifestyle change has always been the recipes that fit in with the principles of the diet. I am sure there are many ways to achieve ketosis and to attain that weight loss goal. However, you do not want to get there by just having the same old dishes over and over again.

Variety is the name of the game here, which is crucial in ensuring the sustainability of the ketogenic diet. With the flavorful and delicious recipes found in this step by step keto cookbook, they will be useful additions for any keto dieter at any stage of their ketogenic journey. I have yet to see anyone complain about having too many easy yet delicious recipes!

ONE LAST THING...

If you enjoyed this book or found it useful, I'd be very grateful if you'd post a short review on Amazon. Your support really does make a difference, and I read all the reviews personally so I can get your feedback and make this book even better.

Thanks, again for your support!

Printed in Great Britain
by Amazon